22 Meditations to Identify and Release Your Fears

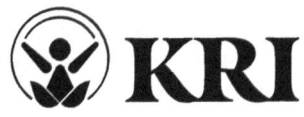

A KUNDALINI RESEARCH INSTITUTE ORIGINAL

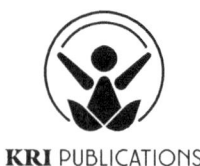

KRI PUBLICATIONS

© 2023 KUNDALINI RESEARCH INSTITUTE
PUBLISHED BY THE KUNDALINI RESEARCH INSTITUTE
TRAINING • PUBLISHING • RESEARCH • RESOURCES
PO BOX 1819
SANTA CRUZ, NM 87532
WWW.KUNDALINIRESEARCHINSTITUTE.ORG
ISBN: 978-0-9639991-9-1

MANAGING EDITOR: MARIANA LAGE (HARISHABAD KAUR)
CONSULTING EDITOR: AMRIT SINGH KHALSA
COVER, CREATIVE CONCEPT AND LAYOUT: FERNANDA MONTE-MÓR
ILLUSTRATOR: JANIS SOUZA
REVIEWER: SIRI NEEL KAUR KHALSA AND DIANA NANU
PROOFREADING: CARLOS ANDREI SIQUARA
EDITORIAL ASSISTANT: ANTONIO LARA SILVA

© **Kundalini Research Institute.** All teachings, yoga sets, techniques, kriyas and meditations courtesy of The Teachings of Yogi Bhajan. Reprinted with permission. Unauthorized duplication is a violation of applicable laws. ALL RIGHTS RESERVED. No part of these Teachings may be reproduced or transmitted in any form by any means, electronic or mechanical, including photocopying and recording, or by any information storage and retrieval system, except as may be expressly permitted in writing by The Teachings of Yogi Bhajan. To request permission, please write to KRI at PO Box 1819, Santa Cruz, NM 87567 or see www.kundaliniresearchinstitute.org.

The diet, exercise and lifestyle suggestions in this book come from ancient yogic traditions. Nothing in this book should be construed as medical advice. Neither the author nor the publisher shall be liable or responsible for any loss, injury, damage, allegedly arising from any information or suggestion in this book. The benefits attributed to the practice of Kundalini Yoga and meditation stem from centuries-old yogic tradition. Results will vary with individuals. Always check with your personal physician or licensed care practitioner before making any significant modification in your diet or lifestyle, to ensure that the lifestyle changes are appropriate for your personal health condition and consistent with any medication you may be taking.

22 Meditations to Identify and Release Your Fears

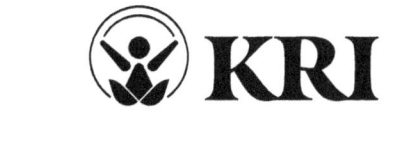

A KUNDALINI RESEARCH INSTITUTE ORIGINAL

SUMMARY

INTRODUCTION 6

BEFORE YOU BEGIN 12
    Tuning In
    Pacing Yourself
    Concluding an Exercise

22 MEDITATIONS TO IDENTIFY AND RELEASE YOUR FEARS

01. Release Fear of Emptiness Within 16
02. Assess Your Fantasies to Release Fear 20
03. Remove Deep Worries and Haunting Thoughts 22
04. Release Fear of Self & Be Yourself 24
05. Conquer Your Fear of Tomorrow 28
06. Eliminate Your Inner Fears 34
07. Assess the Essence of Your Identity and Reality 38
08. Know Your Inner Self and Nurture Emotional Resilience 42
09. Be in the Flow of Present Moment 44
10. Confront Your Dualities and Self-Destructiveness 48
11. Know Your Own Soul 52
12. Conquer Your Animal Aspect and Face the Challenges of Tomorrow ... 56
13. Pituitary Adjustment to Nurture the Capacity to Be Happy 58
14. Develop Your Capacity of Infinity 64
15. Trance Meditation to Refine the Mind 68
16. Self-Blessing To Realize Yourself as a Human Being 72
17. Develop the Capacity to be Infinite 76
18. Cultivate Inner Peace 80
19. Develop Your Presence through the Strength of Your Soul 82
20. Self-Hypnosis to Experience Pratyahar 84
21. Body Adjustment to Eliminate Tension and Stress 86
22. Open to the Unknown and Know Through Intuition 90

INTRODUCTION

It's a well known teaching in Kundalini Yoga that there are two basic energies: fear and love and that, as a polarity, we cannot experience both of them at the same time. In short, whenever there is love, there is no fear and whenever there is fear, there is no love.

Through the practice of Kundalini Yoga physical sets and meditative kriyas, we learn to cultivate love for everything that is, for life itself with all its ups and downs, and to trust the Unknown and relate to Infinity. Bit by bit, we grow within ourselves that space of surrender where we have no doubt that God and we are one, that everything in the Universe is interconnected and that we are part of infinity living a temporary human – finite – experience. Bit by bit, we learn to recognize our fears and let them go. To become fearless, the path is not to radically extirpate all manifestations of fear, but to observe them gently with the neutral mind, so they can be bit by bit dissolved or weakened.

As we all have learned, fear is an instinctive reaction that protects us from what the mind perceives as danger. The problem arises when the patterns and filters of the mind get entangled and confused between what is a potential danger and what is imaginary projection based on past experiences. When we are in fear, we contract, we isolate ourselves from others and ultimately separate ourselves from the world and from the infinite within us. When we are in the flow of love, we feel alive, vivid, expansive, open, all encompassing. This also teaches us something else. In the words of the visionary eighteenth century poet William Blake, "without contraries there is no progression."[1] In order to expand, we need to contract. We shall progress in our expansive experience of love when we live through some form of contraction of fear. In this context, we can understand that fear is not bad in itself. On the contrary, it's indeed necessary as a navigation tool. The key then is to train the mind to assess the fears, acknowledging and afterwards releasing them.

Another inspiring person to bring to the conversation is Martin Luther King Jr., when he reminds us that "Normal fear protects us; abnormal fear paralyzes us. Normal fear motivates us to improve our individual and collective welfare; abnormal fear constantly poisons and distorts our inner lives. Our problem is not to get rid of fear but rather to harness and master it."[2] In a similar tone, analyzing our common human experience with fear, writer and poet Reverend Dave Brown

---

1 BLAKE, William. *The Marriage of Heaven and Hell*. Mineola: Dover Publications, 1994.

2 KING, Martin Luther. *A Gift of Love: Sermons from Strength of Love and Other Preachings*. Boston: Beacon Press, 2012, p. 117.

recalls that "living with, in and through fear must be one of the most enduring of all human experiences throughout our long evolution."[3] He notes that if fear wasn't such a regular companion to humanity, the Bible, for instance, wouldn't be filled with the warning "Fear Not." He claims that it's one of the most common phrases in the holy Christian book – appearing at least 350 times. This, he notes, reinforces how real fear can be in human life, and also how uplifting it is to "fear not!"

Best-selling author and poet Mark Nepo invites us to understand that "Fear is a mood to be moved through, not a voice to be obeyed." He proposes that we can navigate the moments when fear overtake us through the practice of acceptance, tenderness and admiration. "Love moves us toward the miracle, while fear moves us toward the mess. And since fear gets its power from not looking, we are called, no matter our circumstance, to enlist the strength of heart to look through our fears."[4] He also quotes an interesting passage in which the existentialist philosopher Soren Kierkegaard says that a manifestation of anxiety is the "dizziness of freedom." In other words, we sometimes close down or paralyze in the face of the incommensurable expansion that the experience of love brings us.

Because of that, another good way to better deal with fear is to nurture and cultivate love within ourselves. When fear comes, that's when we have to practice, quieting the mind and attuning to our inner self. There seems to be no better way to confront fear each time it appears other than practicing trust in the Unknown. And to enhance our trust in the Unknown, the toolkit we have at our disposal would certainly include breathing exercises, yoga, meditation and inner awareness. Yogi Bhajan reminds us that there is an extra task we should undertake: "We can develop our own caliber. (…) You can have a caliber where you can have depth, width, height and strength."[5]

Since Kundalini Yoga is the Yoga of Awareness, it makes sense that practicing it would lead us towards the confrontation of our fears, to look through our fears and walk away from the paralyzing fear. As we sit to meditate, to do breathing exercises or to work on the physical body and/or the subtle bodies, we gradually build in our minds the capacity to hold the space of the neutral mind to distinguish what is reality and what is illusory, making it easier to let go of the attachments of the ego. As Yogi Bhajan once put it during a

---

3 BROWN, Dave. "Meditations on Fear: Love is but a song to sing, published in Futurist.com (March 14, 2020). Accessible in https://futurist.com/2020/03/22/meditations-on-fear-love-is-but-a-song-to-sing/

4 NEPO, Mark. *The Book of Soul: 52 Paths to Living What Matters*. New York: St. Martin's Press, 2020.

5 Yogi Bhajan, The Library of Teachings, April 5, 1994.

Khalsa Women Training Camp: "The purpose of all yoga is what Kundalini Yoga describes: to become so aware in one's own awareness that the entire creativity of the Creator can be realized and experienced in the finite self. The purpose of Kundalini Yoga is to experience the infinity in the finite self.[6]"

To help us even further in this quest, Yogi Bhajan gave 22 lectures and 22 meditations dedicated to the subject of fears between late 1992 and early 1993. They are mostly dedicated to supporting people to go through the changes and challenging times that marked the transition from the Piscean Age to the Aquarian Age. He mentioned many times in those days that the transition of the ages will bring tremendous fear, feeling of emptiness, numbness, disconnection and internal disruption. To get through the shaky and disruptive time, new internal skills were needed.

In some of these classes, fear was approached indirectly, but always related to how the transition of the ages would impact people and challenge every fiber of their being. In a way, these classes were a preparation for a short run goal – an intense yatra of two weeks to India after a nine year interval[7]. But it was also, ultimately, a long run preparation – the Aquarian Age that would be fully in effect about 21 years after those classes were taught.

A key point that Yogi Bhajan worked throughout these lectures was to reconnect with one's own spirit and own essence as if knowing oneself and cultivating inner awareness were the most important skills required in the Aquarian Age. Lecture after lecture, he provoked the students to just know themselves, to conquer their minds and to strengthen their connection with their souls. In these lectures, fear is qualified as our biggest enemy and also as an animal that hunts us in three dimensional ways: in relation to the past, present and future. Below I selected a few inspiring quotes from these 22 lectures and their respective dates:

» "You will have to survive for being you." *December 1, 1992.*

» "Time has come that you understand the depth of your life (and) that you are master of your own destiny and discipline." *December 3, 1992.*

---

6 Yogi Bhajan, The Library of Teachings, August 12, 1977.

7 This yatra to India happened in March 1993, around 160 members of the community took part in it and was considered an important political and spiritual mission. "We are going there for a special reason, to invoke, to create the theme of joy, happiness and giving people hope, and giving people love and giving people peace of mind." – Yogi Bhajan, March 10, 1993.

- "Basically when it boils down, you have to come to your own self with your own grips. You have to come to grips with your own life." *December 8, 1992.*

- "The highest (form of) therapy is that you should forgive yourself and others. Right on the spot, you should have an attitude of forgiveness." *December 10, 1992.*

- "Kundalini is just to uncoil your reserve energy to live in your total, perfect potential self." *December 15, 1992.*

- "Tomorrow means how much you are facing yourself? How do you carry yourself in life?" (...) "So spirituality is eventually how you face yourself with a smile in life and its confrontation." *December 31, 1992.*

- "I want to make you understand that if you do not know your own soul, you cannot make any goal, and that's why we are suffering." *February 2, 1993.*

- "The exercise which we are teaching you today and this course… The purpose is to train your vitality so that you can face the coming consequences. Sooner or later we have to face the attitude, that is the Age of Aquarius." *February 9, 1993.*

- "You can compete, compare and be confused (or) contain, content and be continuous. Choice is yours." *February 10, 1993.*

- "Humans have to live to a status of a human and you have no human status realized for you." "You got to learn to be consciously intuitive and intuitively stimulating." *February 17, 1993.*

- "The standard is to have the power and guidance of the intuition of the subtle body to find the most subtle remote thing to go for help, serve, elevate, and what that is, is called love!" *February 23, 1993.*

- "The test of life is to be infinite, in being finite and the mind has the capacity to be infinite." *February 23, 1993.*

- » "There is nothing beyond you, there was nothing, there is nothing, and there shall be nothing beyond you. The question is do you connect?" *February 24, 1993.*

- » "Love has no jurisdiction, no territory, no definition (...) Whenever you can define a love, it is not a love. It is your obsession." *March 2, 1993.*

- » "The intention shall only be right, when you have no fear, because when you act under fear, you will act for gain and a loss." *March 2, 1993.*

- » "Kundalini Yoga is a science of life, it is a science of a householder, it is a science of a person who wants to be successful. It is not a 'follow me!' science. No, it won't work. 'Be my student' won't work, because I am my own student. You have to be your own student. You have to practice and experience, and then you have to judge it yourself, with your consciousness." *March 10, 1993.*

The Kundalini Research Institute hopes this new yoga manual can help all Kundalini Yoga practitioners in their exploration of the love and fear polarity, to nurture love within themselves and foster connection with their inner awareness. May these meditations support you further in the journey of assessing your fears, knowing yourself, nurturing your soul and strengthening your intuition. May we all gracefully face the challenges and changes that the Aquarian Age keeps bringing to our lives, attuned to love and increasingly aware of our own fears.

May 2023
Hari Shabad Kaur Khalsa
Mariana Lage
KRI Managing Editor

BEFORE YOU BEGIN

If you're new to Kundalini Yoga, note that it's always a good practice to tune in before you begin your yoga each day. Here we share key points to be aware of when doing the practices below.

Tuning In

Every Kundalini Yoga session begins with chanting the Adi Mantra, **"ONG NAMO GURU DEV NAMO."** By chanting it with the right pronunciation and projection, the student becomes open to their higher self, the source of all guidance, and accesses the protective link between himself or herself and the consciousness of the divine teacher.

Sit in a comfortable cross-legged position with the spine straight. Place the palms of the hands together as if in prayer, with the fingers pointing straight up, and then press the joints of the thumbs into the center of the chest at the sternum. Inhale deeply. Focus your concentration on the Third Eye Point. As you exhale, chant the entire mantra in one breath. If you can't chant on a single breath, then take a quick sip of air through the mouth after "Ong Namo" and then chant the rest of the mantra, extending the sound as long as possible. The sound "Dev" is chanted a minor third higher than the other sounds of the mantra. As you chant, let the sound vibrate the inner chambers of the sinuses and the upper palate to create a mild pressure at the Third Eye Point. The mouth is slightly open and the lips held firm, increasing the resonance while the sound comes out through the nose. Chant this mantra at least three times before beginning your Kundalini Yoga practice.

The "O" sound in Ong is long, as in "go," and of short duration. The "ng" sound is long and produces a definite vibration on the roof of the mouth and the cranium. The "O," as in "go," is held longer. The first syllable of Guru is pronounced as in the word, "good." The second syllable rhymes with "true." The first syllable is short and the second one is long. The word Dev rhymes with "gave".

"Ong" is the infinite creative energy experienced in manifestation and activity. It is a variant of the cosmic syllable "Om," which refers to God in Its absolute or unmanifest state. "Namo" has the same root as the Sanskrit word "Namaste," which means reverent greetings. It implies bowing down. Together, "Ong Namo" means "I call on the infinite creative consciousness," and it opens you to the universal consciousness that guides all action.

"Guru" is the embodiment of the wisdom that one is seeking. "Dev" means higher, subtle, or divine. It refers to the spiritual realms. "Namo," at the end of the mantra, reaffirms the humble reverence of the student. Taken together, "Guru Dev Namo" means, "I call on the divine wisdom," whereby you bow before your higher self to guide you in using the knowledge and energy given by the cosmic self.

Pacing Yourself

Kundalini Yoga exercises may involve rhythmic movement between two or more postures. Begin slowly, keeping a steady rhythm. Then increase gradually, as the body allows, being careful not to strain. Be sure that the spine has become warm and flexible before attempting rapid movements. It is important to be aware of your body and to be responsible for its well-being.

Concluding an Exercise

Unless it says otherwise, an exercise ends by inhaling and suspending the breath for a short time, then exhaling and relaxing the posture. While the breath is being held, apply the Root Lock, contracting the muscles around the anal sphincter, the sex organs, and the Navel Point, while drawing the navel back towards the spine. This consolidates the effects of any exercise and circulates the energy to your higher centers. Hold the breath just beyond a level of comfort. If you experience any discomfort, immediately release the lock and exhale.

"You will have to survive for bein...
come that you understand the de...
master of your own destiny and di...
when it boils down, you have to c...
grips. You have to come to grips w...
"The highest (form of) therapy is t...
others. Right on the spot, you sho...
December 10, 1992. "Kundalini is ...
live in your total, perfect potentia...
means how much you are facing ...
in life?" (...) "So spirituality is even...
smile in life and its confrontation.
you understand that if you do n...
make any goal, and that's why we...

you." December 1, 1992. "Time has
th of your life (and) that you are
pline." December 3, 1992. Basically
ue to your own self with your own
your own life." December 8, 1992.
t you should forgive yourself and
d have an attitude of forgiveness."
st to uncoil your reserve energy to
lf." December 15, 1992. "Tomorrow
urself? How do you carry yourself
ally how you face yourself with a
December 31, 1992. "I want to make
know your own soul, you cannot
e suffering." February 2, 1993.

01 Release Fear of Emptiness Within

December 1, 1992

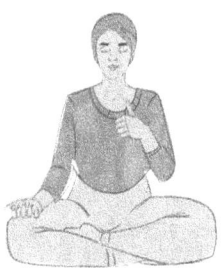

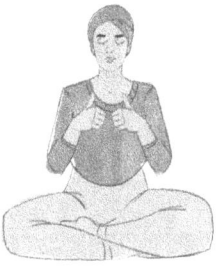

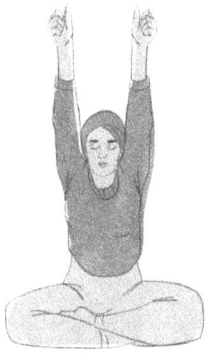

PART ONE
Sit in Easy Pose with a straight spine and apply a light Neck Lock.

Mudra: Rest the right hand on the right knee. Make the left hand into a fist. With the thumb stretched up (maximum stretch some thumbs will curve). Place the fist on the chest over the physical heart.

Eye Focus: Not specified.

Breath: Breath through the nose. Create a steady breath rhythm: The inhalation and suspension of the breath together take **15 seconds** and exhale for **5 seconds**. Each breath is **20 seconds**, 3 breaths per minute.

Time: Continue for **11 minutes (or 33 breaths).**

To End: Make a fist with the right hand with the thumb extended and place it on the right side of the chest, so that both fists are on the chest. Inhale deeply, suspend the breath for **12 seconds**, maintain the mudra and raise the arms straight up and back 8 times; then exhale. Repeat the sequence for a total of 5 breaths. Relax.

Comments: This exercise brings vitality.

PART TWO

Sit in Easy Pose with a straight spine and apply a light Neck Lock.

Mudra: Relax the elbows next to the body, bend the elbows with forearms forward and parallel to the ground, palms down. Lock the Saturn, Sun and Mercury fingers (middle, ring and little fingers) down with the thumbs. Jupiter fingers remain extended and pointing forward. From the elbows, rotate the forearms and hands in small outward circles, simultaneously move the hands away from each other as far as possible, remaining parallel to the ground. Reverse the rotation inward, simultaneously moving the hands to the starting position. Move with force, as fast as possible.

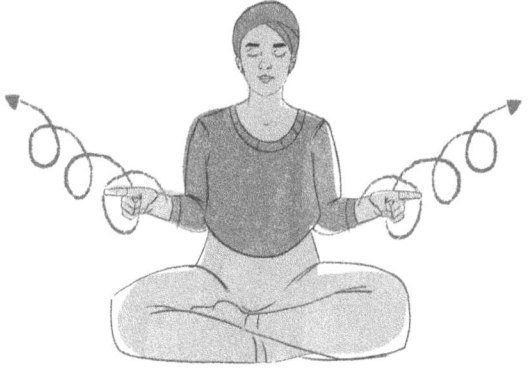

Eye Focus: Not specified.

Breath: Not specified.

Time: Continue for **5 minutes**.

To End: Inhale deeply, suspend the breath for **20 seconds** and squeeze the body from the base of the spine, moving up vertebrae by vertebrae to the base of the skull. Repeat **2 more times**. Immediately begin Part Three.

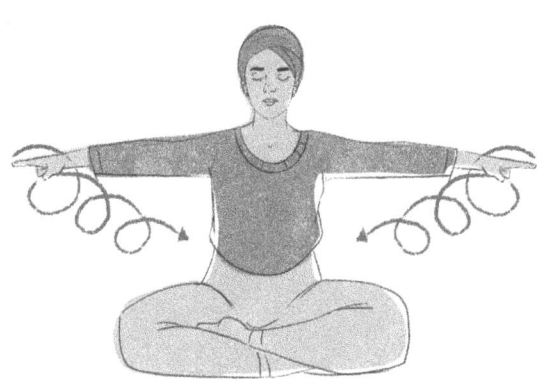

Comments: This exercise is working on the nervous system, on the electromagnetic field.

continue on next page »

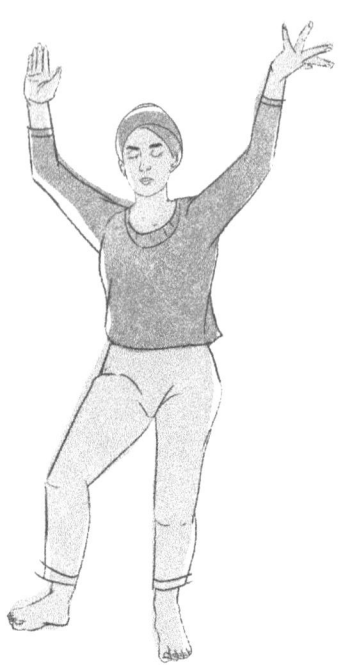

PART THREE
Stand up and dance freely, move the entire body. Focus on moving the shoulders.

Music: Punjabi Drums and Bhangra music were played in the class.

Time: Continue for **31 minutes**. Relax.

Comments: The movement of the shoulders moves the rib cage. This movement affects the circulatory and glandular systems.

"The exercise which we are teaching you today and this course... The purpose is to train your vitality so that you can face the coming consequences. Sooner or later we have to face the attitude, that is the Age of Aquarius." February 9, 1993. "You can compete, compare and be confused (or) contain, content and be continuous. Choice is yours." February 10, 1993.

02 Assess Your Fantasies to Release Fear

December 3, 1992

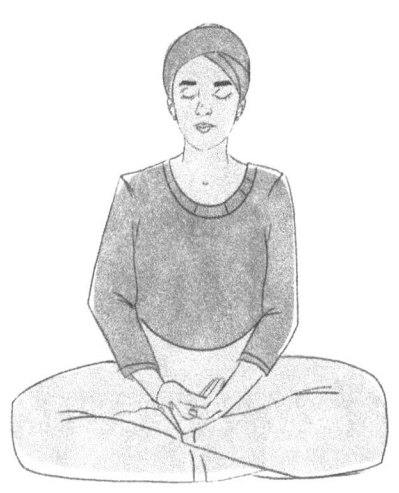

PART ONE

Sit in Easy Pose with a straight spine and apply a light Neck Lock.

Eye Focus: Closed.

Breath: Not specified.

Mental Focus: Be calm and trusting. Bring to mind all of your fantasies. In fantasy, the mind has no barriers. You are both in the non-reality of fantasy and assessing your reality. Penetrate, comparing the two perspectives. Cut through the fear, the weakness. You are within yourself – face the realities of life. Yogis call this process *"pratyahar"* to synchronize through self-processing. If you deny your fantasies and let them go into the subconscious, your life becomes imbalanced from your memory. Thoughts released from your memory change your mood, your mental attitude, your self. If you penetrate and go through it, the metabolism of the body and your aura will change.

Time: 15 minutes.

To End: Begin to yawn. Continue for **1 minute.** Yawning stimulates the vagus nerve and relaxes the brain. Immediately begin Part Two.

PART TWO
Sit in Easy Pose with a straight spine and apply a light Neck Lock.

Mudra: Press the Jupiter (index) finger of the right hand on the Third Eye Point and the Jupiter (index) finger of the left hand on the Heart Center. The other fingers are folded into the hand and the thumbs are extended upwards.

Eye Focus: Closed.

Mental Focus: Connect the two chakras, the Heart Center and Third Eye Point using the knowledge of Jupiter energy. Between those two points bring up your greatest fear. Face it courageously. Don't underestimate your strength. Confront bravely.

Time: 3 ½ minutes.

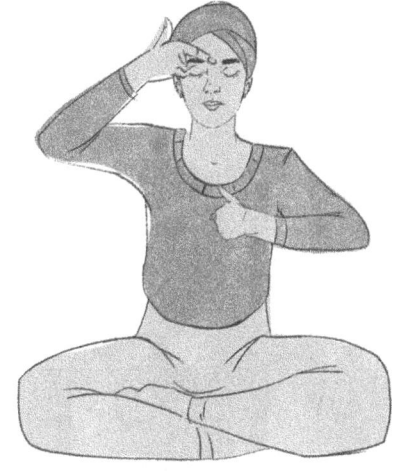

To End: Maintain the mudra, and inhale deeply, suspend the breath for **20 seconds**, squeeze the body; exhale. Repeat 1 more time. Inhale deeply, exhale deeply 2 times. Inhale deeply to your full capacity, suspend the breath for **20 seconds**, tightly squeezing the body; exhale. Relax and talk with each other.

Comments: This meditation kriya releases fears and imagined fantasies.

03 Remove Deep Worries and Haunting Thoughts

December 8, 1992

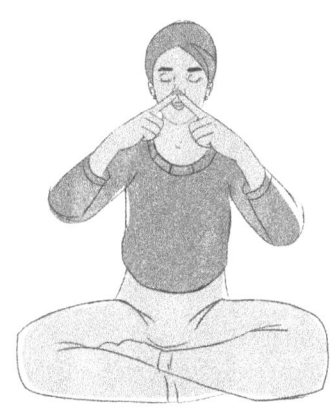

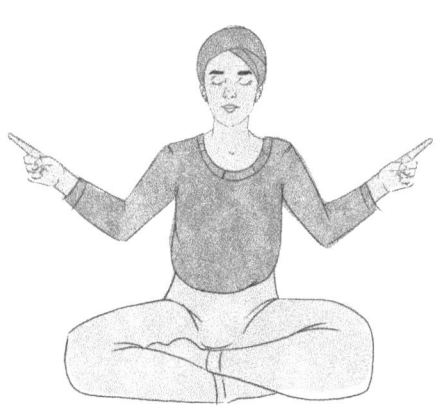

PART ONE

Sit in Easy Pose with a straight spine and apply a light Neck Lock.

Mudra: Make fists with the Jupiter (index) fingers extended and the other fingers held down with the thumbs. Hold the elbows away from the body at Heart Center level and touch the tips of the Jupiter (index) fingers in front of the face. Keep the elbows bent in place and, with a quick powerful movement, open the forearms and bring the hands out to the sides at shoulder level. Instantly the hands spring back to the starting position with the Jupiter (index) fingers touching in front of the face.

Eye Focus: Not specified.

Breath: Inhale, suspend the breath, exhale, 1 or 2 breaths per minute.

Time: 13 minutes.

To End: Inhale deeply, exhale. Immediately move to Part Two.

Comments: Shake fast and hard, and suspend the breath to break through the protective shield and release old memories, the haunting thoughts behind your fears.

PART TWO

Remain in Easy Pose with a straight spine and apply a light Neck Lock.

Mudra: Place the left hand on the Heart Center with fingers pointing to the right, thumb relaxed. With the right elbow close to the body, raise the right hand as if taking a solemn oath, palm facing forward at the level of the shoulder.

Eye Focus: Closed and concentrated on the forehead.

Breath: Breathe very slowly, deeply, suspend the breath and exhale.

Music: Gong was played in the original class (2 beats per second, start with one strike loud, then soft and crescendo to loud, repeat 8 times, then strike hard 8 times).

Time: 9 minutes.

To End: Inhale deeply, suspend the breath for **20 seconds**, exhale, Repeat 1 more time. Inhale deeply, suspend the breath for **20 seconds** and squeeze the right hand as tight as you can, exhale. Relax.

Comments: There is no need to carry the past, it creates problems in your life. Forgive yourself, let go of it. Let the Universe take care of it, and enjoy every moment of life.

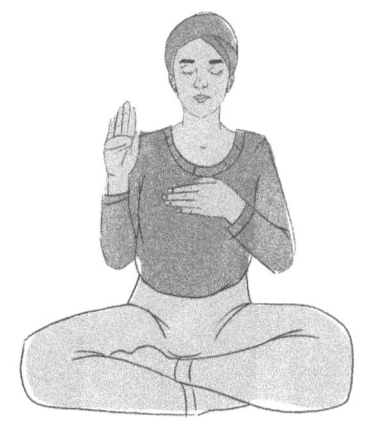

04 Release Fear of Self & Be Yourself

December 10, 1992

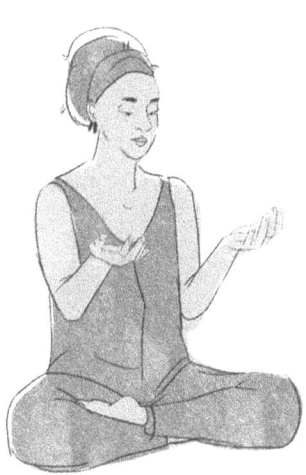

PART ONE

Sit in Easy Pose with a straight spine and apply a light Neck Lock.

Mudra: Brace the elbows at the sides of the body and slightly forward. Bend the elbows, forearms straight forward and raised so that the hands are at the level of the Heart Center. Bend the wrists with relaxed hands and palms facing up. The hands are slightly cupped, ready to receive.

Eye Focus: Look down at the Tip of the Nose. If you see it, focus on the blue pearl, a thin crescent shape.

Breath: Not specified.

Mantra: I AM, I AM NOT. One repetition of the mantra takes 4 seconds with a brief pause between the two phrases. The first phrase sounds like the strike of a gong with the emphasis on AM. There is a brief pause before the second phrase which is a slightly higher pitch with the emphasis on NOT. The mantra vibrates in the skull.

Time: Mentally chant and feel the vibration of the mantra for **12 minutes**. Then chant the mantra out loud for **3 minutes**. Finally, whistle the mantra for **1 minute**. **(16 minutes total)**.

To End: Inhale deeply, suspend the breath for **10 seconds**, exhale. Repeat 1 more time. Inhale deeply, suspend the breath for **20 seconds** and rub every part of the face with both hands, exhale. Relax.

Comments: Magnify the sound within and stabilize the posture, so that you do not fall asleep.

PART TWO

Sit in Easy Pose with a straight spine and apply a light Neck Lock. If practicing with more people, face another person. If doing it alone, imagine you are facing another person.

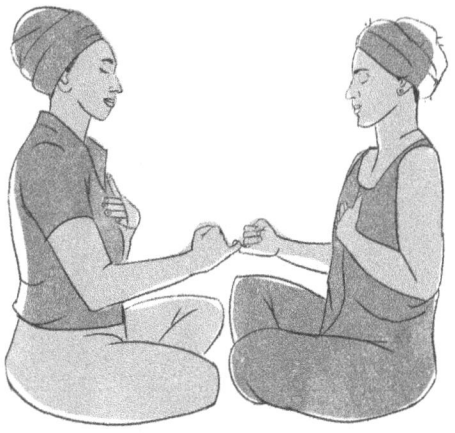

Mudra: Place the left hand on the Heart Center, hook your Mercury (little) finger with the Mercury finger of the other person. Pull as hard as you can.

Eye Focus: Not specified.

Breath: Not specified.

Time: 1 ½ **minutes**.

To End: Relax the posture. Immediately start Part Three.

continue on next page »

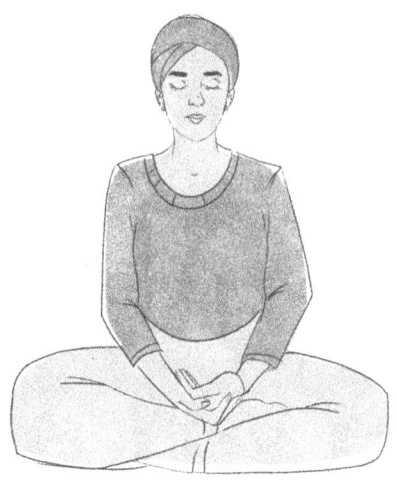

PART THREE
Sit in Easy Pose with a straight spine and apply a light Neck Lock.

Mudra: Relax and meditate.

Eye Focus: Not specified.

Breath: Not specified.

Music: Gong was played in the original class. (Two strikes per second, loudly for 1 ½ second then softly for about 15 seconds, ending with 5 loud strikes and one soft strike).

Time: 2 minutes.

To End: Clap as hard as you can. After 15 seconds, stretch your arms up to 60 degrees with the palms facing forward, hold for **10 seconds**. Keep the arms up and rotate the shoulders forward for **10 seconds**. Keep the arms up and twist the body left and right and move the toes at the same time, continue for **15 seconds**. Relax.

Comments: Fear of the Self limits us. To eliminate this fear, forgive yourself and forgive others. When we are loving, there is no fear. Fear and love cannot coexist.

"Humans have to live to a status of a human and you have no human status realized for you." "You got to learn to be consciously intuitive and intuitively stimulating." February 17, 1993. "The standard is to have the power and guidance of the intuition of the subtle body to find the most subtle remote thing to go for help serve, elevate, and what that is, is called love!" February 23, 1993.

05 Conquer Your Fear of Tomorrow

December 15, 1992

PART ONE
Sit in Easy Pose with a straight spine and apply a light Neck Lock.

Eye Focus: Closed.

Breath: Not specified.

Mental Focus: Call on your consciousness. Ask your consciousness what you would do if a person offers you $1000. Will you accept it, reject it, inquire about it or ignore it? Consciously consider this for **1 ½ minutes**. Answer by repeating the affirmation below.

Affirmation: Never accept and never reject any energy without rationally understanding and intuitively knowing the consequences. Repeat out loud 2 times.

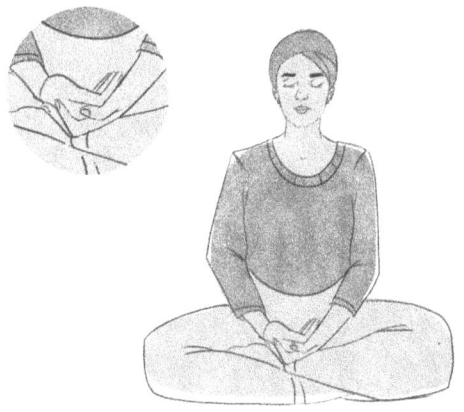

PART TWO
Remain in Easy Pose with a straight spine and apply a light Neck Lock.

Mudra: Interlace the fingers, touch the tips of the thumbs and place the mudra in the lap, palms up. Turn the tongue upside down (the tip of the tongue reaches back under the palate). Suck the tongue and swallow the saliva.

Eye Focus: Closed.

Breath: Not specified.

Time: 3 minutes.

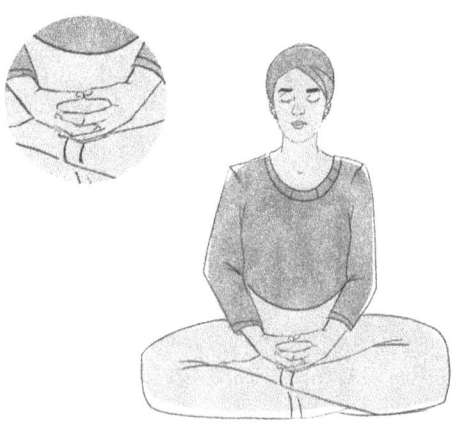

Comments: Use this technique when you are under tremendous stress or fear, and your mouth is dry. You will conquer your fear.

PART THREE

Remain in Easy Pose with a straight spine and apply a light Neck Lock.

Mudra: Touch the fingers of one hand to the corresponding fingers on the opposite hand, with space between them. The palms face each other and are separated, creating a tent shape. Raise the hands in front of the Heart Center, the elbows go out to the sides; there is no bend in the wrist. The fingers point away from the body, the Saturn (middle) fingers point directly forward.

Eye Focus: Closed.

Breath: Full deep breath in 3 parts: inhale, suspend the breath and exhale.

Mental Focus: Breathe consciously. Feel good about each part of your breath. The inhale relates to the future, the suspension to the present and the exhale to the past.

Time: After **3 minutes** of silence, for inspiration, the music "Every Heartbeat" by Nirinjan Kaur was played for **10 minutes**. Total **13 minutes**. Relax and immediately begin Part Four.

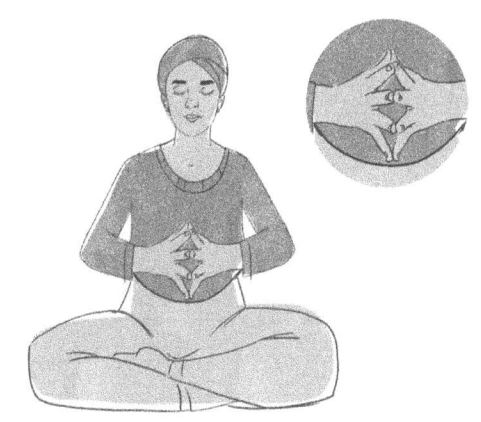

continue on next page »

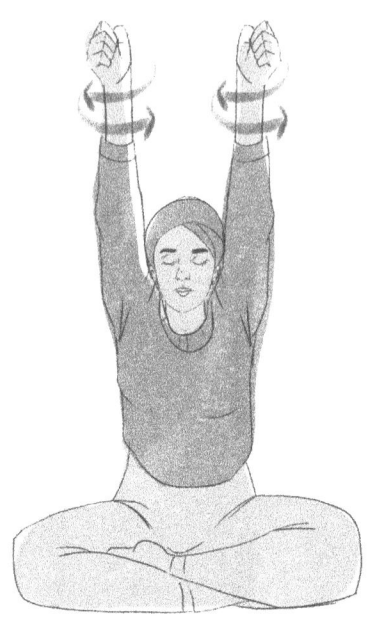

PART FOUR
Remain in Easy Pose with a straight spine and apply a light Neck Lock.

Mudra: Place the tips of the thumbs on the mounds of the Mercury (little) fingers and make tight fists around the thumbs. Raise the arms straight up with no bend or movement in the elbows or wrists. From the shoulders, the arms move in small circles (the left arm moves counterclockwise and right clockwise). Move powerfully from the base of the spine, the entire spine moves; keep the fists tight.

Eye Focus: Not specified.

Breath: Not specified.

Time: 6 minutes.

To End: Inhale deeply, suspend the breath for **10 seconds**, stretch the arms up as high as possible, exhale. Relax.

Comments: Move so powerfully that each vertebra of the spine moves. Even your bottom moves, bringing vitality.

PART FIVE
Remain in Easy Pose with a straight spine and apply a light Neck Lock.

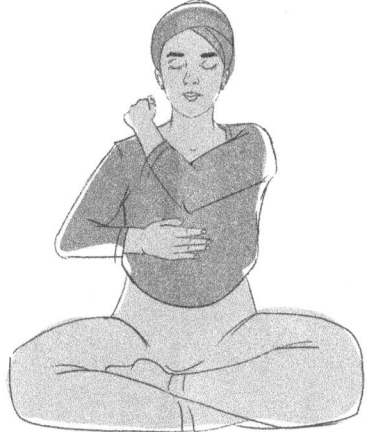

Mudra: Bend the elbows with the hands relaxed in front of the upper abdomen, palms facing the body. Forcefully raise one arm up, bringing hand over the opposite shoulder with palm down. Alternate the arms moving quickly. Feel the pull in the armpits.

Eye Focus: Not specified.

Breath: Not specified.

Time: 1 ½ minutes.
Immediately begin Part Six.

Comments: Done powerfully it brings circulation to the ribcage, chest and throat.

continue on next page »

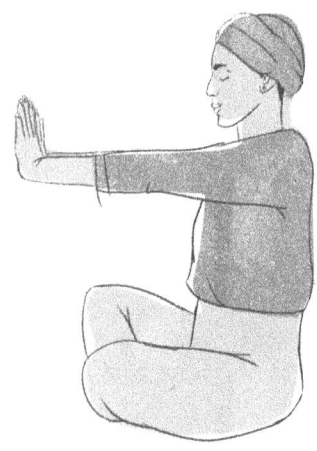

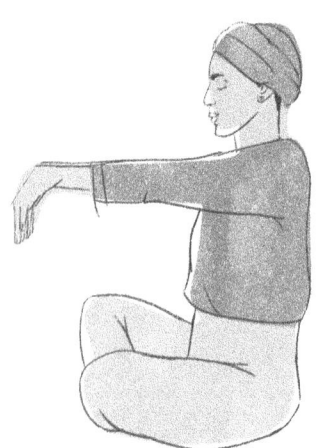

PART SIX

Remain in Easy Pose with a straight spine and apply a light Neck Lock.

Mudra: Stretch the arms forward, parallel to the ground, palms facing down, fingers together. Move the hands rapidly up and down from the wrists. The arms remain steady, only the hands and wrists move.

Eye Focus: Not specified.

Breath: Not specified.

Time: 2 minutes.

To End: Inhale deeply, maintain the arms parallel to the ground, actively pull the arms forward from the shoulders and bend the wrist, palms forward, stretching the hands back as far as possible; suspend the breath for **15-20 seconds**, exhale. Repeat **2 more times**.

The test of life is to be infinite, in being finite and the mind has the capacity to be infinite." February 23, 1993. "There is nothing beyond you, there was nothing, there is nothing, and there shall be nothing beyond you. The question is do you connect?" February 24, 1993. "Love has no jurisdiction, no territory, no definition (...) Whenever you can define a love, it is not a love. It is your obsession." March 2, 1993.

06 Eliminate Your Inner Fears

December 31, 1992

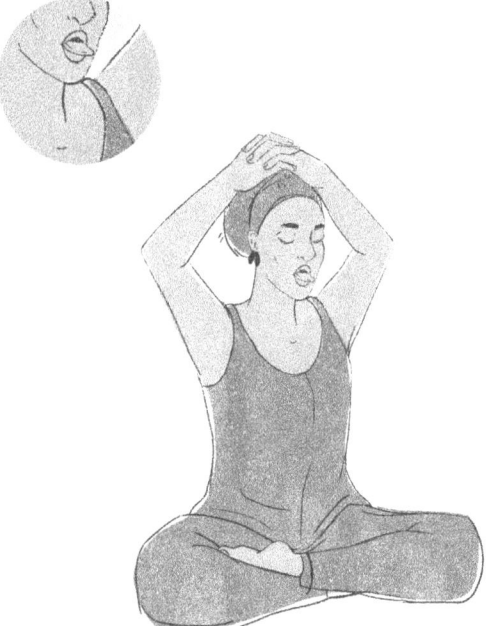

PART ONE
Sit in Easy Pose with a straight spine and apply a light Neck Lock.

Mudra: Interlace the fingers and place the hands on top of the head. Pull the elbows out to the sides, stretching the chest. Hold this posture. Stick out the tongue and quickly move it back and forth in all directions.

Eye Focus: Closed.

Breath: Not specified.

Mental Focus: In the depth of silence, feel the effect within, from the Navel Point to the tongue.

Time: 11 minutes.

Comments: Moving the tongue in this way stimulates the vagus nerve.

PART TWO
Remain in the posture with the tongue moving.

Eye Focus: Closed.

Breath: Breathe deeply through the mouth using the strength of the diaphragm.

Mental Focus: On the exhale, imagine that you are releasing all negativity within the body – physical, mental and emotional.

Time: 5 minutes.

To End: Inhale deeply, suspend the breath for **10 seconds** and exhale. Repeat for 6 more breaths. Inhale deeply, suspend the breath for **20 seconds** and exhale. Repeat for 5 more breaths. On the last breath, suspend as long as possible and exhale with Cannon Breath.

PART THREE
Stand up and dance vigorously, moving your shoulders and keeping your hands higher. (Bhangra Music was played in the class).

Time: 9 minutes.

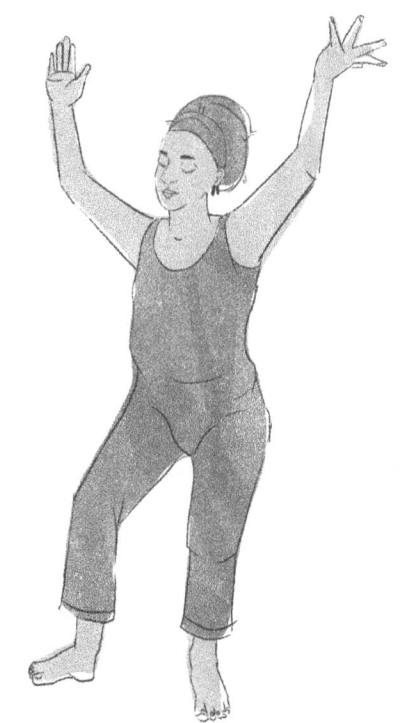

continue on next page »

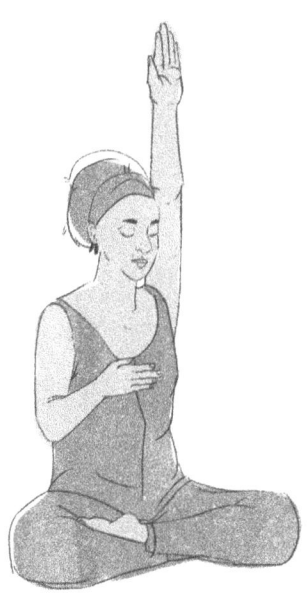

PART FOUR
Sit in Easy Pose with a straight spine and apply a light Neck Lock.

Mudra: Place the left palm on the Heart Center with the fingers pointing to the right. Stretch the right arm straight up perpendicular to the ground. The hand faces forward, fingers pointing up.

Eye Focus: Closed.

Breath: Breathe slowly in three parts. Inhale as long as possible, suspend the breath as long as possible, and exhale as long as possible.

Affirmation: Continuously repeat the word **VICTORY** mentally.

Time: 6-7 minutes.

To End: Inhale deeply, stretch up, tighten the body, suspend the breath for **15 seconds**, and exhale. Relax.

Comments: The word "victory" is powerful. It embodies both your effort and projection. Control the breath and be victorious.

"The intention shall only be right, when you have no fear, because when you act under fear, you will act for gain and a loss." March 2, 1993. "Kundalini Yoga is a science of life, it is a science of a householder, it is a science of a person who wants to be successful. It is not a 'follow me!' science. No, it won't work. 'Be my student' won't work, because I am my own student. You have to be your own student. You have to practice and experience, and then you have to judge it yourself, with your consciousness."

07 Assess the Essence of Your Identity and Reality

January 5, 1993

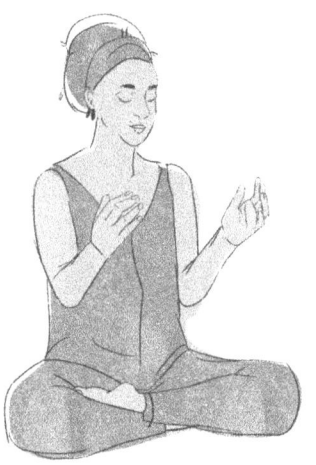

PART ONE

Sit in Easy Pose with a straight spine and apply a light Neck Lock.

Mudra: Rest the elbows lightly against the body, bring the forearms forward parallel to each other. Raise the forearms until the hands are at the level of the upper chest. The palms face each other and the fingers are slightly apart and curved.

Eye Focus: Not specified.

Breath: Slow, complete Long Deep Breath.

Mental Focus: Become calm and tranquil. Concentrate on your skin. From the inside out, feel your physical boundary. Touch your skin mentally, not with your hands. Feel your existence, your territory. Know the boundary of yourself, your physical body. Feel your own boundary.

Time: 9 minutes.

Comments: When you are aware of your own physical boundaries, you know the essence of your identity and reality. Then you can be aware of others' boundaries.

PART TWO

Remain in Easy Pose with a straight spine and apply a light Neck Lock.

Mudra: Place the left hand on the Heart Center, fingers together and pointing to the right. Stretch the right arm straight forward and up at a 60-degree angle. The hand extends forward, palm flat, fingers together. There is no bend in the elbow or wrist.

Eye Focus: Closed.

Breath: Conscious breath.

Mental Focus: Having felt and acknowledged the boundary of the body in Part One, now allow the Universe to provide whatever is lacking; fill the emptiness. Bring in health, happiness, prosperity, respect, love, and fulfill yourself. After **5 minutes**, maintain the posture and begin to mentally chant the Mantra of the Aquarian Age. As you mentally chant the Aquarian March, feel your victory. Victory of the soul; victory over time; victory over death. Achieve victory.

Mantra:
SAT SIREE, SIREE AKAAL
SIREE AKAAL, MAAHAA AKAAL
MAAHAA AKAAL, SAT NAAM
AKAAL MOORAT, WHAA-HAY GUROO

continue on next page »

Time: Continue **6 minutes** in silence, and **5 more minutes** mentally chanting the mantra. (Musical version "The Aquarian March," by Nirinjan Kaur was played in the original class.) Total of **11 minutes**.

To End: Inhale deeply, stretch the arm as far as you can, suspend the breath for **15 seconds**, exhale. Inhale deeply and exhale through the mouth. Inhale deeply, tighten the body, stretch the arm, suspend the breath for **10 seconds**, exhale. Inhale deeply, stretch the arm and press the left hand on the Heart Center to create balance, suspend the breath for **15 seconds**, exhale and repeat one more time suspending the breath for **30 seconds**. Relax.

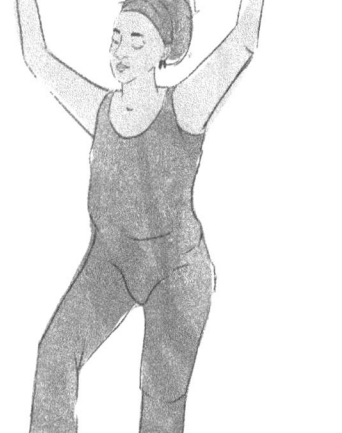

PART THREE
Stand up and dance vigorously, moving your shoulders and keeping your arms high. (Bhangra Music was played in the class).

Time: 9 minutes.

You will have to survive for being you." December 1, 1992. "Time has come that you understand the depth of your life (and) that you are master of your own destiny and discipline." December 3, 1992. Basically when it boils down, you have to come to your own self with your own grips. You have to come to grips with your own life." December 8, 1992. "The highest (form of) therapy is that you should forgive yourself and others. Right on the spot, you should have an attitude of forgiveness." December 10, 1992.

08 Know Your Inner Self and Nurture Emotional Resilience

January 7, 1993

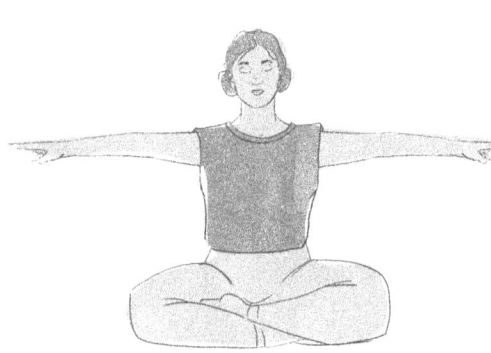

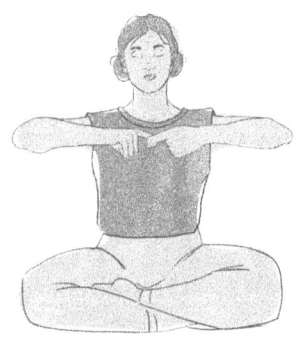

Sit in Easy Pose with a straight spine and apply a light Neck Lock.

Mudra: Make fists with both hands, Jupiter (index) fingers extended and the other fingers held down with the thumbs. Stretch the arms to the sides parallel to the ground, fists facing down. Keeping the elbows straight, rotate the arms from the shoulders, rapidly in small circles, up and backward. The circles are no more than 9 inches (23 cm) in diameter.

Eye Focus: Not specified.

Breath: Breath of Fire.

Time: 7 minutes.

To End: Maintain the mudra and interlock the Jupiter (index) fingers at the level of the shoulders with the arms parallel to the ground. Inhale deeply, suspend the breath for **10 seconds**, forcefully pull on the Jupiter fingers, and exhale. Repeat **4 more times**. On the last breath, exhale with Cannon Fire, suspend the breath out for **20 seconds**, pull on the Jupiter fingers with a great deal of strength, and inhale. Remain seated, relax and talk with each other for a few minutes. If practicing alone, talk to yourself out loud.

Comments: Practicing this meditative kriya supports healing the health of your organs. Discomfort indicates improper diet, lack of exercise, or lack of emotional resilience.

"Kundalini is just to uncoil your reserve energy to live in your total, perfect potential self." December 15, 1992. "Tomorrow means how much you are facing yourself? How do you carry yourself in life?" (...) "So spirituality is eventually how you face yourself with a smile in life and its confrontation." December 31, 1992. "I want to make you understand that if you do not know your own soul, you cannot make any goal, and that's why we are suffering." February 2, 1993.

09 Be in the Flow of Present Moment

January 12, 1993

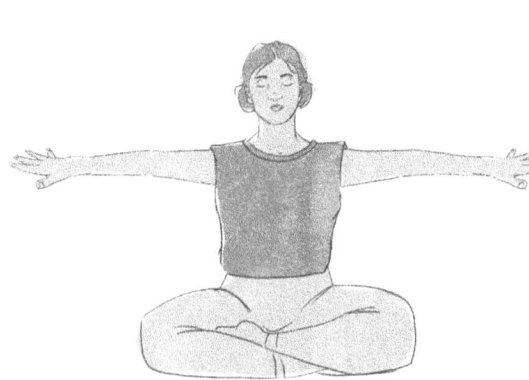

PART ONE
Sit in Easy Pose with a straight spine and apply a light Neck Lock.

Mudra: Extend the arms out to the sides, parallel to the ground, palms facing down. Make fists with both hands, thumbs on the outside. Forcefully open palms with tense fingers spread apart and then relax the hands back into fists. Move rapidly keeping the arms parallel to the ground, only the hands move. The opening outward motion is powerful.

Eye Focus: Tip of the Nose.

Breath: Not specified.

Time: 11 minutes.

To End: Maintain the posture with the hands in fists. Inhale deeply, suspend the breath for **15 seconds**, stretching the arms to the sides and Cannon Fire exhale. Repeat **2 more times**. Relax for several minutes.

PART TWO

Sit in Easy Pose with a straight spine and apply a light Neck Lock.

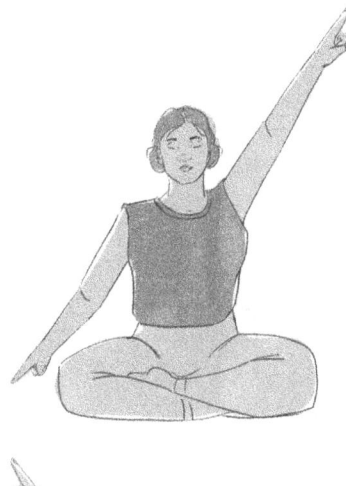

Mudra: Make fists with both hands, with the Jupiter (index) fingers extended and the other fingers held down with the thumbs. Extend the arms out to the sides, parallel to the ground, palms facing down. Keeping the arms stretched, lower one arm until the Jupiter finger touches the ground while the other arm raises up to maintain a straight diagonal line across the body. Alternate the arms moving up and down. Move fast, 90 times per minute.

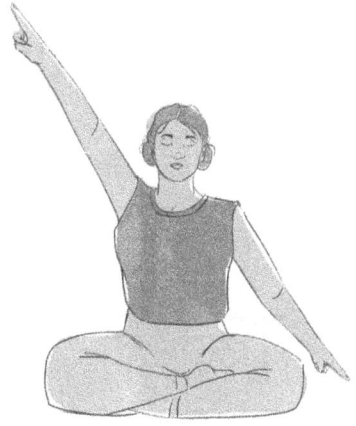

Eye Focus: Not specified.

Breath: Not specified.

Time: 7 minutes.

To End: Maintain the posture with the arms at a diagonal. Inhale deeply, suspend the breath for **10-15 seconds**, twist to the side with the raised arm, stretch as much as you can and exhale. Repeat **2 more times**. Relax for a few minutes.

Comments: This exercise is beneficial for breast and heart health.

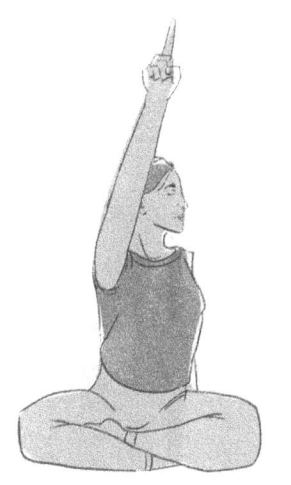

continue on next page »

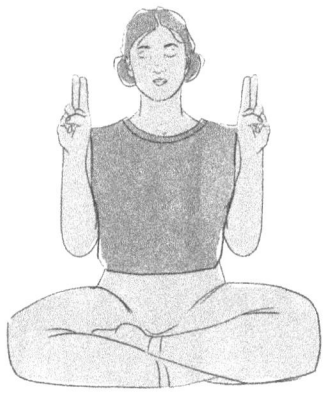

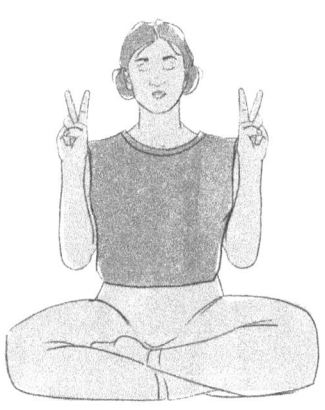

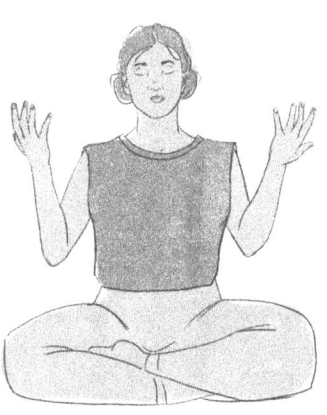

PART THREE
Sit in Easy Pose with a straight spine and apply a light Neck Lock.

Mudra: Make fists with both hands, with the Jupiter (index) and Saturn (middle) fingers extended and the other fingers held down with the thumbs. Relax the elbows at the sides of the body, raise the forearms up perpendicular to the ground, palms face forward with no bend in the wrists. The Jupiter and Saturn fingers point straight up. Rhythmically, spread the Jupiter and Saturn fingers apart and close them. The motion of the two fingers is precise and conscious. Nothing else moves.

Eye Focus: Not specified.

Breath: Not specified.

Time: 4 ½ minutes.

To End: Inhale deeply, suspend the breath for **15 seconds**, open fists and rapidly move the hands, twisting from the wrists, Cannon Fire exhale. Repeat **2 more times**. Relax, stretch and talk with others or to yourself for a few minutes.

"The exercise which we are teaching you today and this course... The purpose is to train your vitality so that you can face the coming consequences. Sooner or later we have to face the attitude, that is the Age of Aquarius." February 9, 1993. "You can compete, compare and be confused (or) contain, content and be continuous. Choice is yours." February 10, 1993.

10 Confront Your Dualities and Self-Destructiveness

January 30, 1993

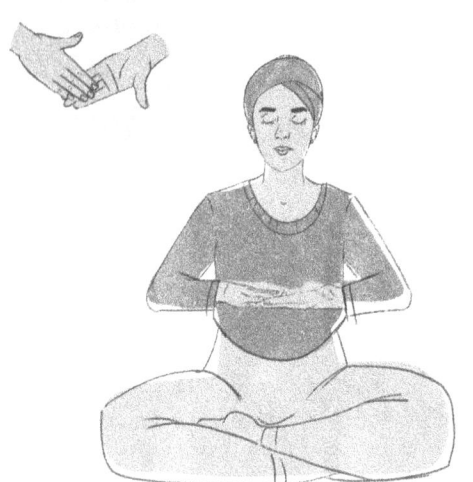

PART ONE

Sit in Easy Pose with a straight spine and apply a light Neck Lock.

Mudra: Hold the hands in front of the body between the Solar Plexus and Heart Center level, the elbows are away from the body. The left hand faces up and the right hand faces down with the fingers together and thumbs stretched away from the fingers. Place the right fingers on top of the left fingers at a 90-degree angle. The thumbs and hands create a zigzag pattern. Move the hands up and down ½-1 inch (1-2.5 cm). Keep the hands and thumbs stiff. Maintain a steady rhythm throughout the exercise.

Eye Focus: Closed, look at the Moon Center (tip of the chin).

Breath: Not specified.

Mental Focus: Concentrate on the fingers touching each other and the balance of the movement of the hands. Be alert, the body will want to stop, but keep moving.

Time: 27 minutes.

Comments: This exercise works on the pituitary gland and gives the stamina to keep up rather than give up.

PART TWO

Remain in Easy Pose.

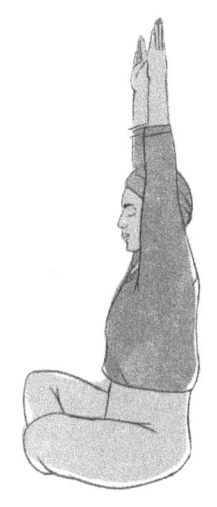

Mudra: Stretch the arms straight up, hands facing forward. From the Heart Center, shoulders, neck and wrists, dip down and come forward and up in a wave-like motion.

Eye Focus: Not specified.

Breath: Inhale deep as the arms stretch up, exhale as the body dips down.

Time: 13 ½ minutes.

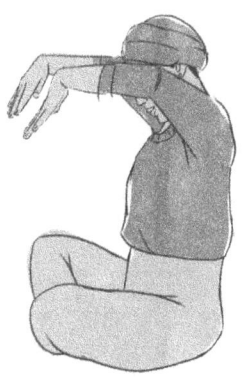

To End: Inhale deeply, stretch the arms up, spread the fingers wide, suspend the breath for **15 seconds**, and exhale. Repeat **2 more times**. Come out of the posture, stretch the body for **1 minute**; then relax for a few minutes.

Comments: This challenging exercise works on your glandular and nervous systems to maintain your vitality. You may mentally sing any song to help you keep up.

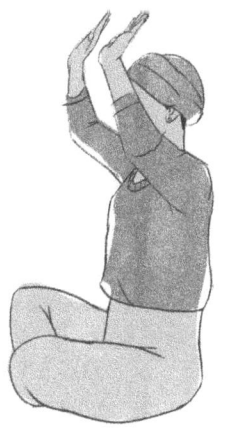

continue on next page »

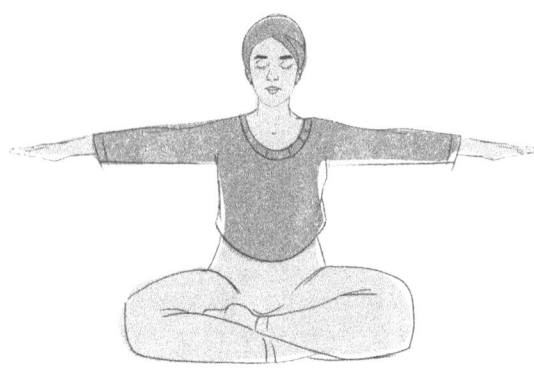

PART THREE
Sit in Easy Pose with a straight spine and apply a light Neck Lock.

Mudra: Stretch the arms out to the sides at shoulder level, parallel to the ground, palms facing down. Move the arms forward 60 degrees and back to the starting position. There is no bend in the elbows. The entire body from the base of the spine moves. The rhythm is one cycle per second.

Eye Focus: Not specified.

Breath: Not specified.

Time: 9 minutes.

Comments: This exercise is excellent for the circulatory system.

PART FOUR
Lie on your back in Corpse Pose.

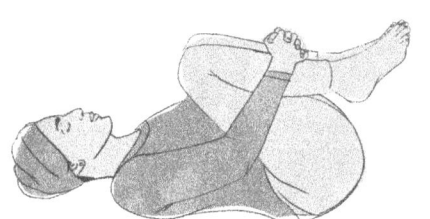

Mudra: Bring the knees into the chest, heels touching the buttocks. Wrap the arms around the legs, interlace the fingers and hold the knees to the chest; lock the position tight.

Eye Focus: Closed.

Music: Gong was played in the class. (2 strikes per second, starting gently softly and gradually increasing the sound to moderately loud. End with one or two stronger strikes.)

Time: 7 minutes.

To End: Slowly wake up, stretch each part of the body for **1 minute**. Immediately begin Part Five.

PART FIVE
Remain in Corpse Pose.

Mental Focus: Mentally relax every part of your body, from your toes, heels, feet, ankles, up to your face, lips, teeth, tongue, nose, cheeks, eyes, eyebrows, your entire head, hair, and internally all of your organs and muscles and bones. Continue for **2-3 minutes**.

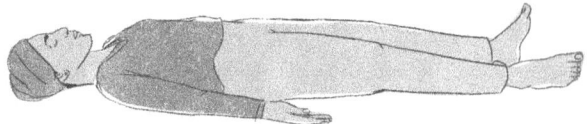

Visualization: Imagine you are a large bird like an eagle. Leave the body, fly high towards the sun. Continue for **1 minute**. Then take your time and slowly descend and come back to the body. Take **1 minute**.

Total Time: 4-5 minutes.

To End: Do Cat Stretch to both sides.

11 Know Your Own Soul

February 2, 1993

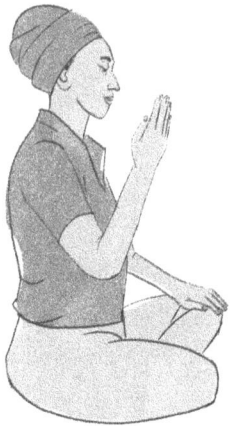

PART ONE
Sit in Easy Pose with a straight spine and apply a light Neck Lock.

Mudra: Rest your right elbows at the side of your body. Raise the right hand up at a 30-degree angle from the body in front of the shoulder, palm facing the body and fingers together. There is no bend in the wrist. Left arm relaxed in a comfortable position.

Eye Focus: Turn your head to look down your nose and gaze on the wrist.

Breath: Inhale through the nose and Cannon Fire exhale into the center of the hand.

Music: ANG SANG WAA-HAY GUROO (A version by Nirinjan Kaur was played in the class in a low volume).

Time: 22 minutes.

To End: Inhale deeply, suspend the breath for **15 seconds**, exhale. Immediately begin Part Two.

Comments: Maintain a powerful breath throughout the exercise to release tension.

PART TWO
Remain in Easy Pose with a straight spine and apply a light Neck Lock.

Mudra: Place the left hand on the Heart Center with fingers pointing to the right, thumb relaxed. With the right elbow close to the body, raise the right hand as if taking a solemn oath, palm facing forward at the level of the shoulder.

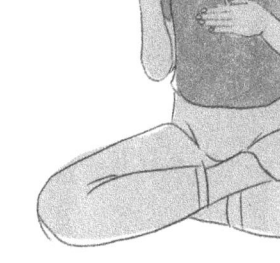

Eye Focus: Closed.

Breath: Slow, complete, Long Deep Breath.

Music: Continue to listen to the mantra **ANG SANG WAHE GURU** for **3 minutes**. Then listen and mentally repeat the mantra "Bountiful, Blissful, Beautiful" for **11 minutes** (The musical version by Nirinjan Kaur was played in the original class). Play the music loud and feel it in the heart.

**I AM BOUNTIFUL, BLISSFUL
AND BEAUTIFUL
BOUNTIFUL, BLISSFUL AND
BEAUTIFUL I AM
EK ONG KAAR SATGUR PRASAAD
ANAND BHAYAA MAYREE MAA-AY
SATIGUROO MAI PAA-YAA
SATIGUROO TAA PAA-YAA
SEHEJ SAYTEE
MAN VAJEEAA VAADHAAEEAA
RAAG RATAN PARVAAR PAREEAA**

continue on next page »

8 Mantra translation: "I am bountiful, blissful, and beautiful. Bountiful, blissful and beautiful I am. Creator and Creation are One. By the Grace of the True Guru. I am in ecstasy, O my Mother, for I have found my True Guru. I have found my True Guru, with intuitive ease, and my mind vibrates with the music of bliss. The jeweled melodies and celestial harmonies have come to sing the Shabd. The Lord dwells within the minds of those who sing the Shabad, the Word. Says Nanak, I am in ecstasy, for I have found my True Guru."

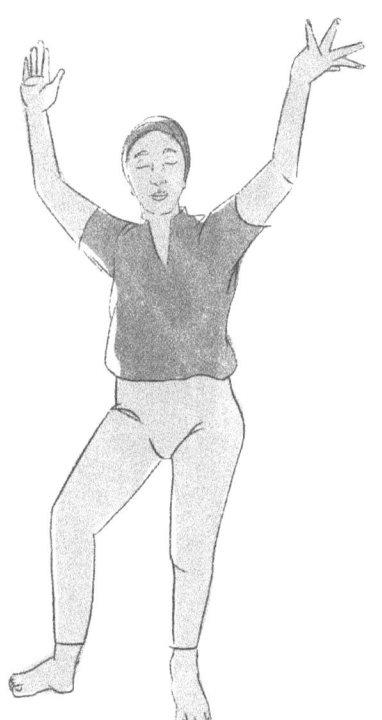

**SHABD GAAVAN AAEEAA
SHABDO TAA GAAVHO HAREE
KAYRAA MAN JINEE VASAA-YAA
KAHAI NAANAK ANAND HOAA
SATIGUROO MAI PAA-YAA**[8]

Affirmation: For the first **3 minutes**, mentally focus on the affirmation "I am the light within me and around me." Then, for the last **11 minutes**, focus on the lyrics of the song, "I am the light of my soul. I am bountiful, I am beautiful, I am bliss."

Time: 14 minutes.

To End: Inhale deeply, stretch the arms straight up, fingers wide, tighten and stretch the body upward, suspend the breath for **20 seconds**; Cannon Fire exhale. Repeat **2 more times**. In the last cycle, pull the navel in and stretch higher. Relax for a few minutes.

Comments: As you relax in this exercise, befriend your soul.

PART THREE
Stand up and dance vigorously, moving your shoulders and keeping your arms high. (Bhangra Music was played in the original class).

Time: 17 minutes.

PART FOUR

Sit in Easy Pose with a straight spine and apply a light Neck Lock.

Mudra: Make fists with the Jupiter (Index) fingers extended and the other fingers held down with the thumbs, bend the elbows and point the Jupiter fingers up, hands facing each other at the level of the face. Make backward and outward small circles with the Jupiter fingers, move the wrists, move very fast, vigorously, so powerful that the body jumps from the floor.

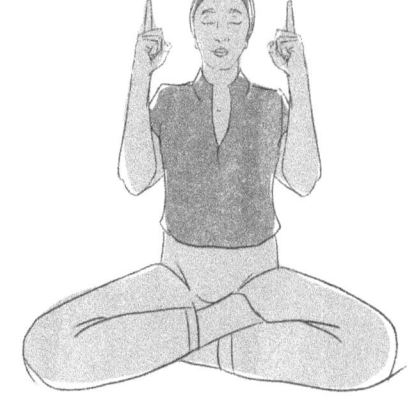

Eye Focus: Not specified.

Breath: Not specified.

Time: 4 minutes.

To End: Inhale deeply, suspend the breath **5-10 seconds**, place the left hand on the Heart Center and the right hand on top, press very hard, exhale through the mouth. Repeat **2 more times**. Relax.

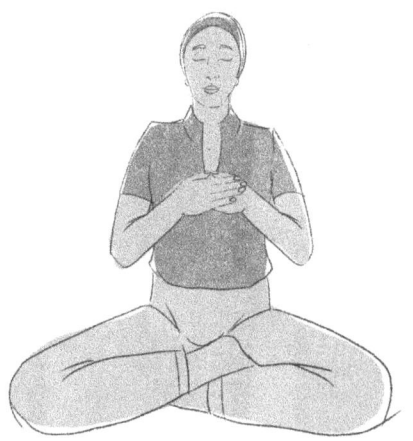

Comments: This exercise promotes the health of the glandular system, the liver, and the pancreas.

12 Conquer Your Animal Aspect and Face the Challenges of Tomorrow

February 3, 1993

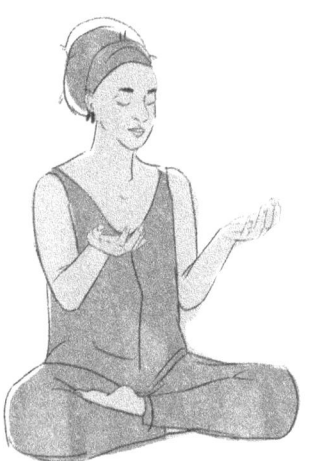

PART ONE

Sit in Easy Pose with a straight spine and apply a light Neck Lock.

Mudra: Place the elbows at the sides of the body. Bend the elbows, bring forearms straight forward and up, so that the hands are at the level of the Heart Center. Palms facing up, bend the wrists with relaxed hands. Fingers relaxed apart and hands slightly cupped, ready to receive.

Eye Focus: Through the closed eyes, concentrate at the 2 points on the hairline in line with the center of each eyebrow.

Breath: Slow, complete, Long Deep Breath.

Mantra: After **14 minutes**, the mantra **ANG SANG WAHE GUROO** was played in the original class.

Time: 19 minutes.

To End: Inhale deeply, suspend the breath for **5-10 seconds**, squeeze the body, exhale. Repeat **2 more times**.

Comments: This meditation controls your animal nature to develop the mind, the brain and physical body to have the vitality to face the changing times. You will not be content trying to control the environment, but rather by controlling the self.

"Humans have to live to a status of a human and you have no human status realized for you." "You got to learn to be consciously intuitive and intuitively stimulating." February 17, 1993. "The standard is to have the power and guidance of the intuition of the subtle body to find the most subtle remote thing to go for help, serve, elevate, and what that is, is called love!" February 23, 1993.

13 Pituitary Adjustment to Nurture the Capacity to Be Happy

February 9, 1993

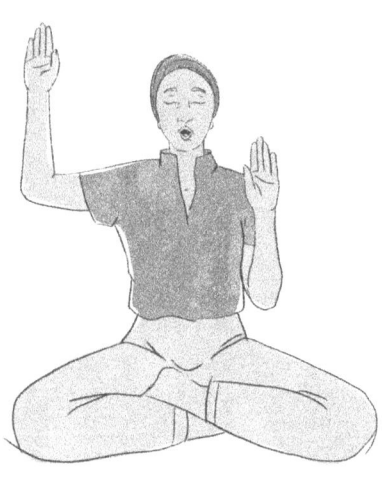

PART ONE

Sit in Easy Pose with a straight spine and apply a light Neck Lock.

Mudra: Relax the left elbow at the side of the body and raise the forearm straight up. The hand is at shoulder level facing forward with the fingers together and thumbs relaxed. Raise the right arm out to the side, upper arm parallel to the ground and raise the forearm straight up perpendicular to the upper arm. The hand faces forward with the fingers together and thumbs relaxed. There is no bend in the wrists.

Eye Focus: Not specified.

Breath: Inhale powerfully through the nose, exhale powerfully through "O" mouth. Each breath takes about 1 second.

Time: 3-11 minutes.

To End: Inhale deeply, suspend the breath for **10 seconds**, stretch the arms up straight, palms forward and shake the hands from the wrists; exhale. Relax for **1 minute**.

PART TWO

Remain in Easy Pose with a straight spine and a light Neck Lock.

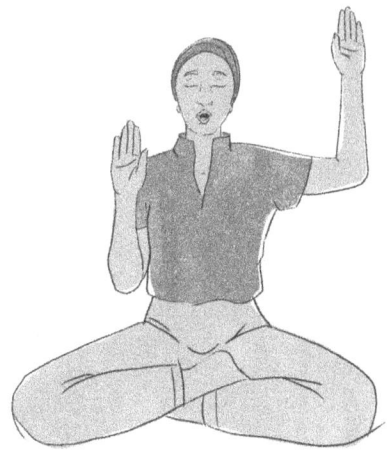

Mudra: Same posture as Part One with the arms reversed. Relax the right elbow at the side of the body and raise the forearm straight up. The hand is at shoulder level facing forward with the fingers together and thumbs relaxed. Raise the left arm out to the side, upper arm parallel to the ground and raise the forearm straight up perpendicular to the upper arm. The hand faces forward with the fingers together and thumbs relaxed. There is no bend in the wrists.

Eye Focus: Not specified.

Breath: Inhale powerfully through the nose, exhale powerfully through "O" mouth. Each breath takes about 1 second.

Time: 3-11 minutes.

To End: Inhale deeply, suspend the breath for **10 seconds**, stretch the arms up straight, palms forward and shake the hands quickly from the wrists; exhale. Relax for **1 minute**.

Comments: Parts 1 and 2 are a balance of the hemispheres of the brain and increase vitality.

continue on next page »

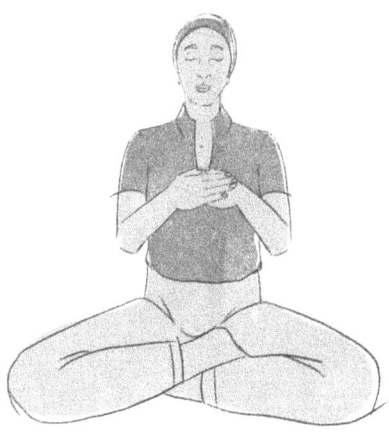

PART THREE
Remain in Easy Pose with a straight spine and a light Neck Lock.

Mudra: Place the left hand on the Heart Center and the right hand on top of the left hand. Press hard on the Heart Center.

Eye Focus: Not specified.

Breath: Inhale deeply through the nose, exhale completely through "O" mouth. Each breath takes about **5 seconds**.

Time: 3-11 minutes.

To End: Inhale deeply for **5 seconds**, suspend the breath for **10 seconds**, stretch the arms up straight, palms forward and shake the hands quickly from the wrists; exhale. Immediately begin Part Four.

PART FOUR
Remain in Easy Pose with a straight spine and a light Neck Lock.

Mudra: Raise the right elbow out to the side and place the right hand on the forehead, with the four fingers together pointing to the left and the thumb relaxed. Place the left hand on the navel.

Eye Focus: Closed.

Breath: Not specified.

Music: Gong was played in the original class – it starts softly, gradually becoming louder then soft again repeating several times.

Mental Focus: Meditate, leave the body and fly towards the sun. Merge with the waves of the gong. Continue for **7 minutes**.

Visualization & Affirmation: Imagine your spine like a tube of light. Purify your body. Mentally repeat: "**HEALTHY AM I, HAPPY AM I, HOLY AM I, HEALTHY AM I, HAPPY AM I, HOLY AM I, HEALTHY AM I, HAPPY AM I, HOLY AM I. HEALTHY AM I, HAPPY AM I, HOLY AM I. I AM BEAUTIFUL, BOUNTIFUL, BLISSFUL.**" Continue for **2 minutes**.

Time: 9 minutes total.

continue on next page »

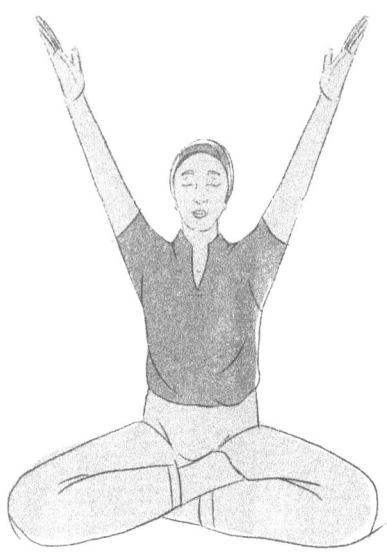

PART FIVE
Remain in Easy pose with a straight spine and a light Neck Lock.

Mudra: Stretch the arms up to 60 degrees with no bend in the wrists, the hands are relaxed and face each other with the fingers together and thumbs relaxed. The hands are in a receptive posture.

Eye Focus: Closed.

Breath: Not specified.

Visualization: Receive the energy of the heavens through your hands and allow it to circulate throughout your body. The breath gives life and all that we need to be happy.

To End: Inhale deeply, suspend the breath a couple of seconds and exhale. Relax for a few minutes.

Time: 3-11 minutes.

PART SIX

Remain in Easy Pose with a straight spine and a light Neck Lock.

Mudra: Firmly clap the hands in front of the chest.

Eye Focus: Not specified.

Breath: Not specified for **30 seconds**. Stick the tongue out and breathe through the mouth (Dog Breath) for **30 seconds**. Whistle a song for **1 minute**. (In the original class, the national anthem was whistled).

Time: 2 minutes total.

Comments: After practicing this kriya, to seal its effect, drink 6-8 ounces of milk with ½ teaspoon of ground black pepper that has been warmed to a boil.

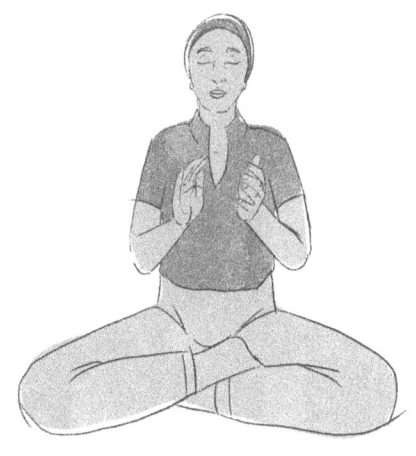

14 Develop Your Capacity of Infinity

February 10, 1993

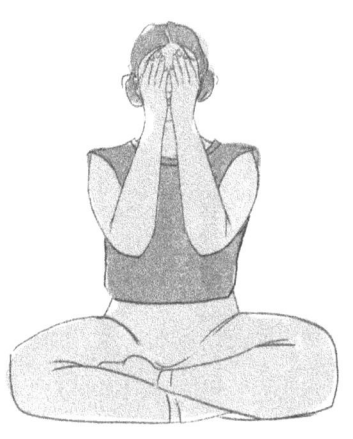

PART ONE

Sit in Easy Pose with a straight spine and apply a light Neck Lock.

Mudra: Place the elbows at the sides of the body and raise the forearms in front of the body parallel to the ground with the hands relaxed and face up, fingers pointing away from the body. There is no bend in the wrists. Inhale as you raise both hands up to cover the eyes, exhale as you return the arms to the starting position. It is important to maintain a steady rhythm.

Eye Focus: Open, looking straight ahead.

Breath: Powerful breath. Inhale deeply through the nose for **2-3 seconds**, exhale through the "O" mouth for **2-3 seconds.**

Time: 8 minutes.

To End: Inhale deeply, interlock the hands, stretch the arms straight up with palms down and lean back as far as possible. Suspend the breath for **10 seconds**, exhale. Repeat **2 more times**. Relax for a few minutes.

PART TWO

Sit in Easy Pose with a straight spine and apply a light Neck Lock.

Mudra: Raise forearms perpendicular to the ground and parallel to each other. The hands face the body at the face level. Cross the hands in front of the face, right hand closer to the body. The hands pause as you exhale into the palms and return to the starting position on the inhale. The breath must be forceful so that you feel the warmth of the breath on the palm.

Eye Focus: Open, looking straight ahead.

Breath: Inhale deeply through the nose, exhale powerfully through the "O" mouth. A complete breath takes **2-3 seconds**.

Time: 5 minutes.

To End: In the starting position with palms forward, inhale deeply, suspend the breath for **15-20 seconds** and vigorously shake the hands in all directions, move quickly, exhale. Repeat **2 more times**. Relax for a few minutes.

Comments: This exercise removes tension and stress from previous incarnations.

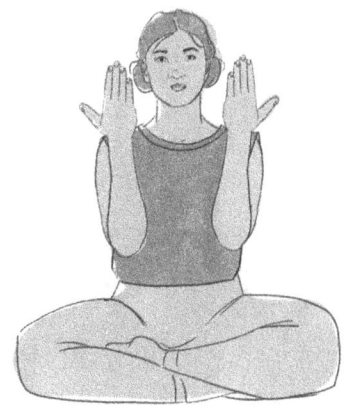

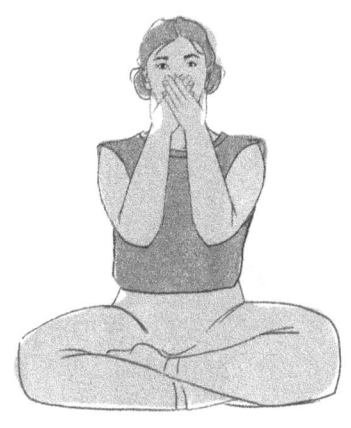

continue on next page »

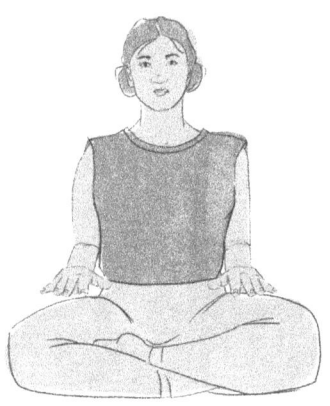

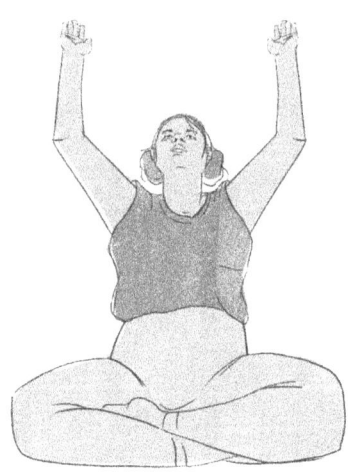

PART THREE
Sit in Easy Pose with a straight spine and apply a light Neck Lock.

Mudra: Reach the arms forward parallel to the ground with a slight bend in the elbows; palms face the ground with fingers relaxed forward. Inhale, from the diaphragm, lift the chest up and arch backwards. Simultaneously raise the arms up until the elbows, still bent, are a little higher and wider than the shoulders. The forearms reach up and back. The head stays aligned with the neck. Exhale as you return to the starting position.

Eye Focus: Not specified.

Breath: Inhale through the nose and forcefully exhale through the "O" mouth.

Time: 3 minutes.

To End: Inhale deeply, stretch backward as far as you can, chest out and chin in, squeeze the body, suspend the breath for **10 seconds**, exhale. Repeat **2 more times**. Relax and sing a song for **1 ½ minute**, if you are in a group everyone sings the same song. Immediately begin Part Four.

Comments: "Without potential, you have no power; without vitality, you have no virtues; without doing, you have no experience"– Yogi Bhajan.

PART FOUR

Remain in Easy Pose with a straight spine and a light Neck Lock.

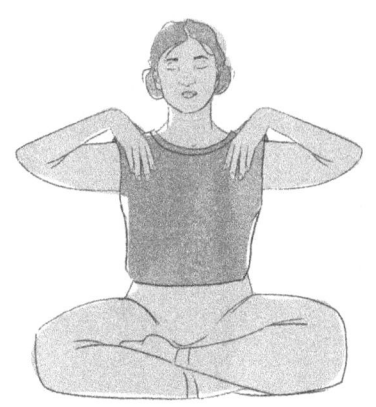

Mudra: Grasp the shoulders with the fingers in front, thumbs in back. The elbows stretched to the sides and upper arms parallel to the ground.

Eye Focus: Closed.

Breath: Not specified.

Mental Focus: Leave the body and like a bird fly to the moon. (Gong was played in the original class. Gong started with 1 medium loud strike, a short pause, then 7 waves from soft to loud. Started at 1 hit per second, increased to 2 hits per second and ended in 30 seconds of strong fast hits a short pause and 1 final strong loud hit).

Time: 5 minutes.

To End: Inhale deeply, squeeze the body tight, try to lift the body from the buttocks, suspend the breath for **20 seconds**, Cannon Fire exhale. Repeat **2 more times**. Relax.

15 Trance Meditation to Refine the Mind

February 16, 1993

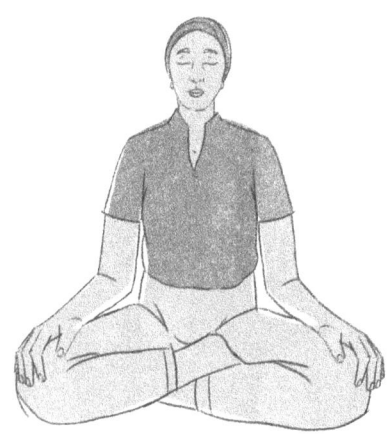

There are no breaks between the parts of this meditation.

Sit in Easy Pose with a straight spine and apply a light Neck Lock.

Mudra: There is no specified hand mudra. In your seated posture, relax the body from the toes, feet, legs, buttocks, up the body, the hands, shoulders, neck, chin and face. Remain relaxed.

Eye Focus: Closed.

Breath: Long, slow deep breath.

a) For **2 minutes**, look down to the center of the Earth. Go deeper and deeper into the core of the Earth.

b) Mentally repeat and listen to the inner sound "I am gud God, I am relaxed." Note use the short vowel sound so that the word GOOD becomes GUD. Continue for **12 ½ minutes**.

c) Continue to mentally repeat and listen to the inner sound: "I am gud God, I am relaxed," as a musical version of the mantra **KAAL AKAAL SIREE AKAAL MAHAA AKAAL, AKAAL MOORAT WHAA-HAY GUROO** is played in the background. Continue for **3 minutes**.

d) Mentally chant the mantra **KAAL AKAAL SIREE AKAAL MAHAA AKAAL, AKAAL MOORAT WHAA-HAY GUROO** for **17 ½ minutes** as you follow the guided meditation below:

Let yourself go, don't resist. Go beyond your comfort and discomfort, rise and fall, leave it to God. Go. With hope and promise, stand face to face before the bright white light of God. Let yourself go. Go beyond mentally holding and resisting. Your body will not like to let go. It feels like losing life. There is a war between being alive and being dead. Let it go, let it go. The mind doesn't like it at all, so there is great tension; a great conflict between you and what you are doing. The reality is that there is always a conflict between you and your doing. That's a hidden reality, it's subconscious living. Because of this conflict, you do secret things, things which are non-realistic. Pray to deathlessness. Rise and resurrect into the form of light. In healing rise, rise, rise. You cannot tolerate an enemy nor a friend. The question is not about enemy or friend; it is about tolerance. To tolerate is to be totally right. Expand; give your mind width, focus on a light like a sun and give it a width and keep on reciting the mantra. You always give your mind length never width. Without width you are handicapped. Heal yourself. (For the last **4 minutes**, play the gong along with the music.)

e) For **1 ½ minutes**, mentally repeat and listen to the inner sound: "I am gud God, I am relaxed."

Total Time: 36 ½ minutes.

To End: Inhale deeply for **5 seconds**, suspend the breath for **15 seconds**, exhale for **10 seconds**. Repeat **2 more times**. The last time as you suspend the breath, squeeze every muscle of the body, gather all of the energy and Cannon Fire exhale.

Comments: Self-created sound is very potent. Listening to the inner sound, your intuition opens. 'Man jeetai jag jeet.' Conquer your mind and you conquer the world. As you repeat this mantra, it becomes inscribed in your memory. Your mind and body may react. Allow whatever happens to happen, don't resist it. In this part, the background music relaxes the body, as you continue to listen to the mantra you create within you. Do nothing but focus on the mantra you are creating against the background music.

The following simple warm-up is suggested before doing this meditation: Stretch your limbs and every part of the body for **30 seconds**. Sit in Easy Pose with a straight spine and apply a light Neck Lock. Flex the spine, the fingers and toes for **15 seconds**. Do each of the next movements for **5 seconds** – roll the eyes, circle the tongue in the mouth, and raise and lower the shoulders. Next, the right hand grasps the left hand in front of the Heart Center, with the elbows out to the sides and the forearms parallel to the ground. Press as hard as possible for **10 seconds**. Maintain the pressure and draw the navel in for another **5 seconds**.

The test of life is to be infinite, in being finite and the mind has the capacity to be infinite." February 23, 1993. "There is nothing beyond you, there was nothing, there is nothing, and there shall be nothing beyond you. The question is do you connect?" February 24, 1993. "Love has no jurisdiction, no territory, no definition (...) Whenever you can define a love, it is not a love. It is your obsession." March 2, 1993.

16 Self-Blessing To Realize Yourself as a Human Being

February 17, 1993

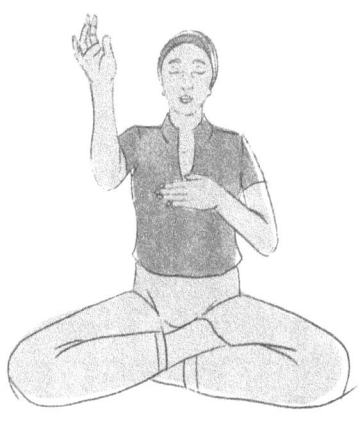

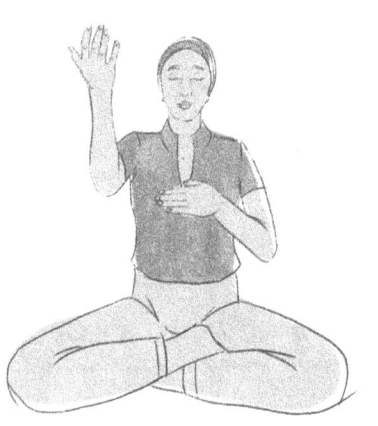

PART ONE

Sit in Easy Pose with a straight spine and apply a light Neck Lock.

Mudra: Place the left hand at the Heart Center with the fingers pointing towards the right and the thumb relaxed apart. Raise the right arm up with the elbow slightly lower and wider than the shoulder. Bring the forearm forward and bend the elbow so that the hand is at the level of the top of the head. The hand and fingers are very relaxed, palm facing forward. From Mercury (little) finger, the hand moves in and up in a curved motion, as if lifting something to infinity and quickly returns to starting position. The arm does not move, only the hand moves. Remain very relaxed and maintain a constant rhythm.

Eye Focus: Closed.

Breath: Not specified.

Mental Focus: Relax and release. Let yourself go. Let go of your existence.

Time: 13 minutes.

PART TWO
Remain in Easy Pose.

Mudra: Bend forward bringing the forehead to the ground; relax the shoulders and the entire body.

Eye Focus: Closed.

Breath: Initially take 3 deep breaths and then breathe naturally.

Time: 2 minutes.

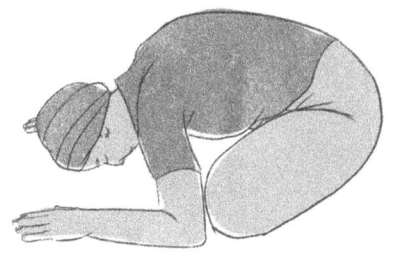

PART THREE
Come sitting up in Easy Pose.

Mudra: Move every part of your body in ways that you do not normally move.

Eyes: Closed.

Breath: Not specified.

Time: 2 minutes.

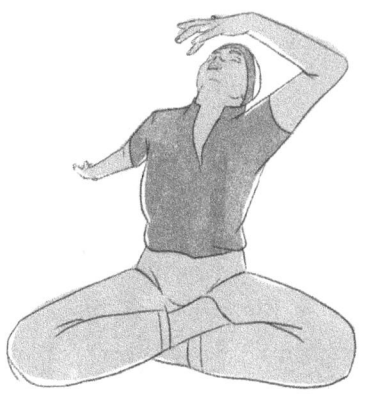

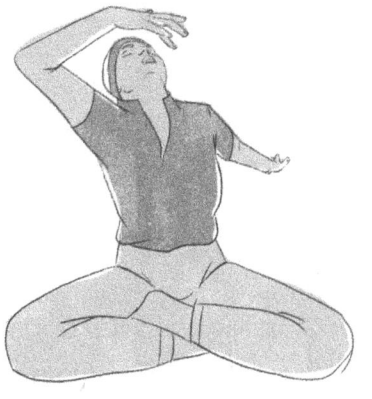

continue on next page »

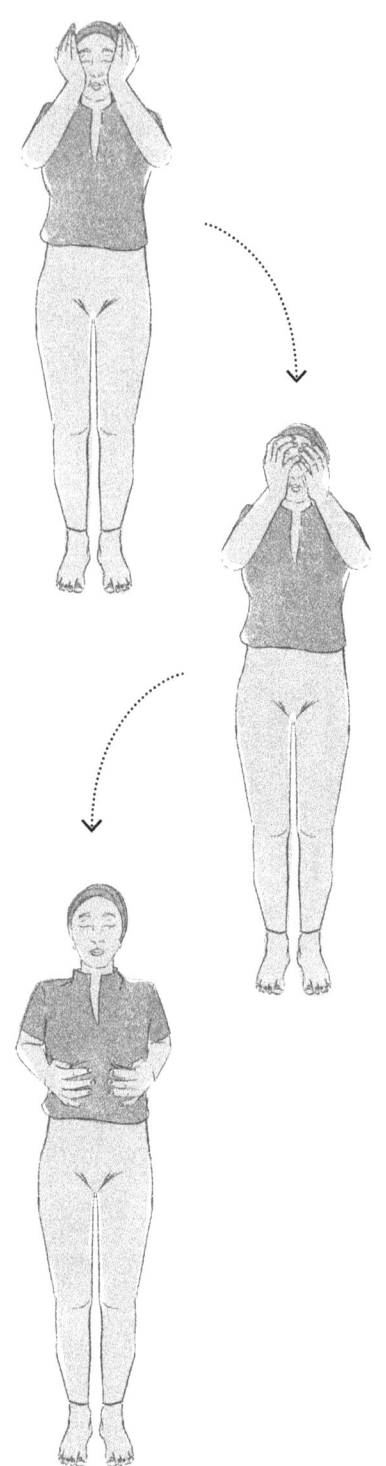

PART FOUR
Stand up.

Mudra: Massage the under the cheek bones to the ears with the heel of the palms. Continue for **1 ½ minutes**. Massage the entire face for **1 minute**. Place the palms on the ribcage just below the breast on the 7th rib, massage the area, moving the ribcage for **1 minute**.

Eye Focus: Closed.

Breath: Not specified.

Time: 3 ½ minutes total.

"The intention shall only be right, when you have no fear, because when you act under fear, you will act for gain and a loss." March 2, 1993. "Kundalini Yoga is a science of life, it is a science of a householder, it is a science of a person who wants to be successful. It is not a 'follow me!' science. No, it won't work. 'Be my student' won't work, because I am my own student. You have to be your own student. You have to practice and experience, and then you have to judge it yourself, with your consciousness."

17 Develop the Capacity to be Infinite

February 23, 1993

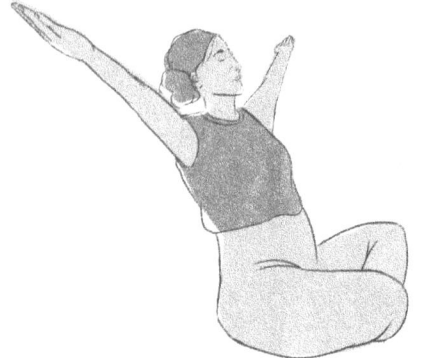

PART ONE
Sit in Easy Pose with a straight spine and apply a light Neck Lock.

Mudra: Extend the arms out to the sides and up about 30 degrees. The elbows are straight with the palms facing up. Keep the spine straight, lift the lower spine and lean back as far as possible, stretching the diaphragm area. Keep a balance with the arms.

Eye Focus: Closed.

Breath: Not specified.

Time: 3-11 minutes.

To End: Inhale deeply, suspend the breath for **10 seconds,** interlock the fingers, stretch the arms up and away from the body, exhale. Relax.

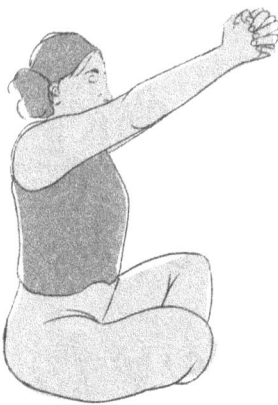

PART TWO
Sit in Easy Pose with a straight spine and apply a light Neck Lock.

Mudra: Extend the arms out to the sides at shoulder height with the hands stiff and palms facing down. Keep the elbows straight and move the arms up and down like a bird's wings. Move from the shoulders.

Eye Focus: Not specified.

Breath: Not specified.

Time: 11 minutes.

To End: Inhale deeply, suspend the breath for **10 seconds**, interlock the fingers, stretch the arms up and away from the body, exhale. Relax.

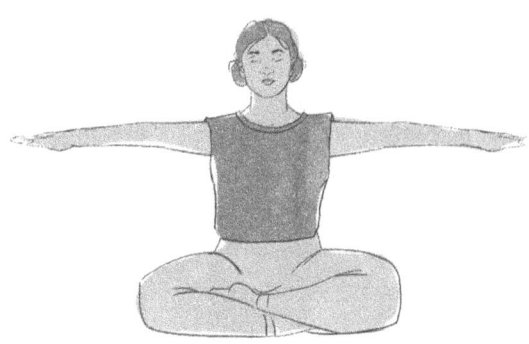

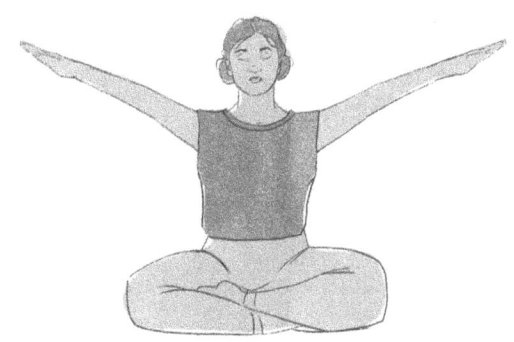

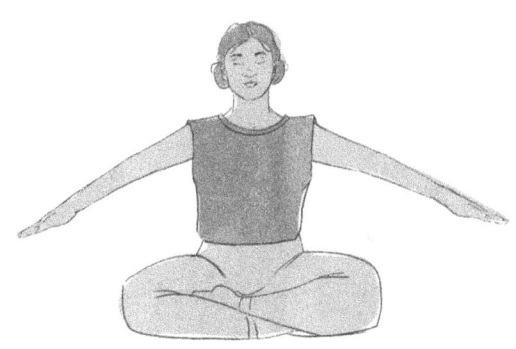

continue on next page »

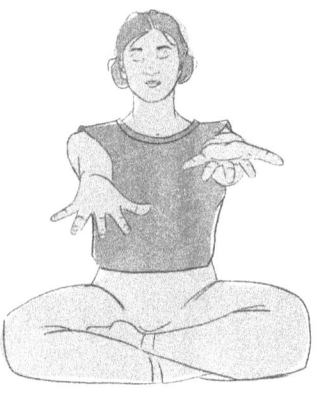

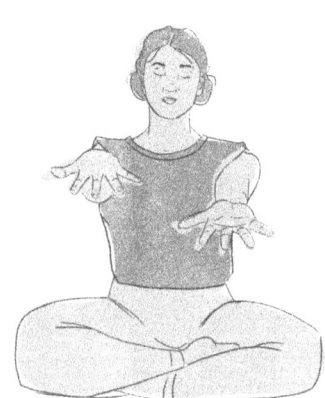

PART THREE
Sit in Easy Pose with a straight spine and apply a light Neck Lock.

Mudra: Extend the arms straight forward parallel to the ground and to each other. The fingers are spread wide, the right hand faces down and left hand faces up. Keep the elbows stretched forward. Tilt the head back, without collapsing the back of the neck. The arms rise **6-8 inches (15-20 cm)** and return to the starting position. As one arm rises, as the other descends. Move rapidly.

Eye Focus: Tip of the Nose.

Breath: Not specified.

Time: 3 minutes.

To End: Inhale deeply, suspend the breath for **10 seconds**, interlock the fingers, stretch the arms up and away from the body, exhale. Relax.

Comments: If you feel dizzy during this exercise stop immediately.

PART FOUR

Sit with the legs extended forward.

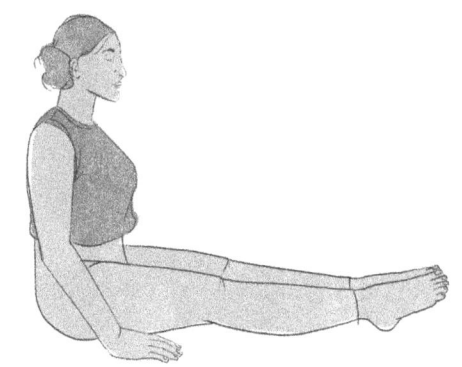

Mudra: Stretch the toes forward as far as you can. After **1 minute**, extend the arms forward and raise the legs, in seated Stretch Pose Variation. Continue for **1 minute**.

Eye Focus: Not specified.

Breath: Not specified.

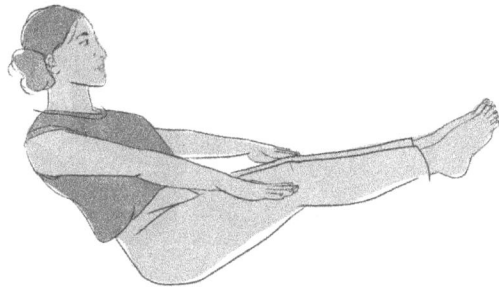

Comments: Part Four is essential to balance the meridian points and the energy flow in the body.

18 Cultivate Inner Peace

February 24, 1993

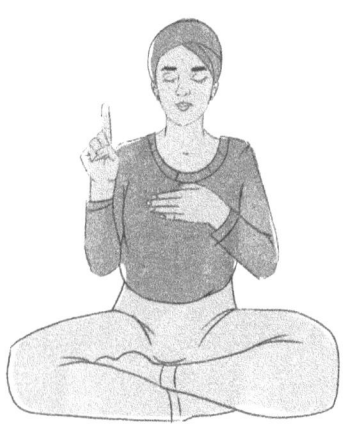

PART ONE

Sit in Easy Pose with a straight spine and apply a light Neck Lock.

Mudra: Place the left hand on the Heart Center with the fingers pointing to the right, thumb relaxed. Make fist with the right hand, Jupiter (index) finger extended and the other fingers held down with the thumb. Bring the right elbow to the side of the body, bend the elbow, with the forearm perpendicular to the ground, palm facing forward and the Jupiter finger pointing straight up. Turn the tongue and press the upper palate strongly with the back of the tongue. Sit steady as if you are the most divine being.

Eye Focus: Tip of the Nose.

Breath: Not specified.

Music: After **3 minutes**, listen to the instrumental Ardas Bhaee for **11 minutes**, "Liberation," by Wahe Guru Kaur for **5 minutes** and finally "Rakhe Rakhanahar," by Singh Kaur for **10 minutes**.

Time: 29 minutes.

To End: Inhale deeply, suspend the breath and pump the navel for **10 seconds**, exhale. Repeat 1 more time. Then inhale deeply, suspend the breath for **5-10 seconds** and pump the navel; exhale, suspend the breath for **15 seconds** and continue pumping the navel. Repeat **2 more times**. Relax, talk with each other about worldly things for about **10 minutes**.

Comments: When we are getting in and out of stress, the body and mind feel uneasy. This period is called the twilight zone. This exercise will eliminate years of stress.

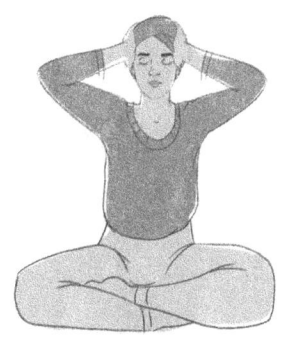

PART TWO

Sit in Easy Pose with a straight spine and apply a light Neck Lock.

Mudra: Place the base of your palms on the temples with the fingers pointing back; press with maximum strength for **1 minute**. Without pausing, lower the hands over the ears and press as hard as you can for **1 minute**.

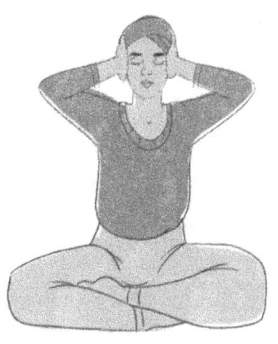

Eye Focus: Closed.

Breath: Not specified.

Mantra: Sing loudly the slow version of Long Time Sun song.

Time: 2 minutes.

To End: Place both hands at the Heart Center and mentally pray for **30 seconds**.

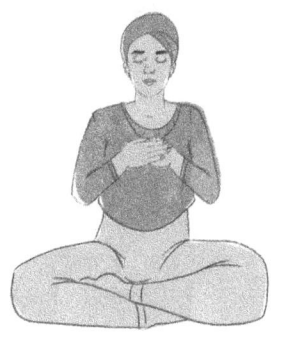

19 Develop Your Presence through the Strength of Your Soul

March 2, 1993

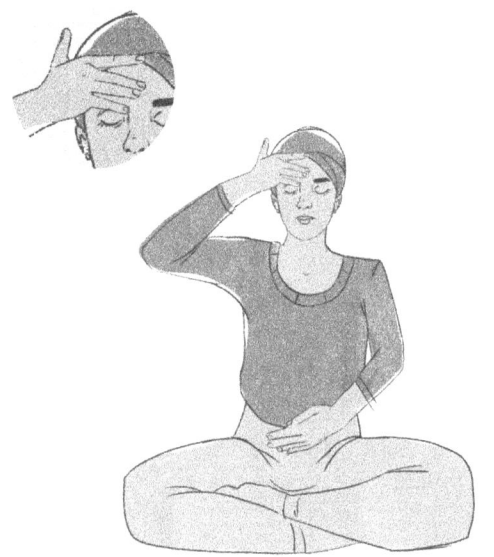

PART ONE
Sit in Easy Pose with a straight spine and apply a light Neck Lock.

Mudra: With the Sun (ring) and Saturn (middle) fingers of the right hand together and the other fingers relaxed apart, raise the right arm, elbow to the side, and place the pads of those two fingers on the Third Eye Point. The other fingers do not touch the body. Place the left palm on the Navel Point, with the fingers pointing towards the right. Sit light and elevated by lifting the ribcage so that there is no weight or pressure on the liver and other abdominal organs. Hold this posture steady and straight.

Eye Focus: Closed.

Breath: Not specified.

Music: "God Is Within Me," by Nirinjan Kaur Khalsa was played in the class. Sing for the last **5 ½ minutes**.

GOD IS WITHIN ME.
I'M DWELLING WITHIN THEE.
I HAVE NO FEAR, I SEE GOD CLEAR:
GOD IN ALL, BIG AND SMALL.
I HAVE NO FEAR, I SEE GOD CLEAR:
GOD IN ALL, BIG AND SMALL.
GOD IS WITHIN ME, ME AND GOD ARE ONE.
I'M DWELLING WITHIN THEE, GOD AND ME ARE ONE.
AS THE MOON AND SUN, SHINING ON EVERYONE.
ONE GOD ABOVE ALL,
GOD IN ALL, BIG AND SMALL.
EVERY PROBLEM OF FEAR IS SOLVED.
GOD IN ALL, BIG AND SMALL.
EVERY PROBLEM OF FEAR IS SOLVED.

CHATTR CHAKKR VARTEE, CHATTR CHAKKR BHUGATAY
SUYUMBHAV SUBHANG SARAB DAA SARAB JUGTAY
DUKAALANG PRANAASEE DAYAALANG SAROOPAY
SADAA UNG SUNGAY ABHANGANG BIBHOOTAY

Time: 22 minutes.

To End: Inhale deeply, and exhale. Inhale deeply, suspend the breath for **10-15 seconds**, squeeze the body, and exhale. Repeat **1 more time**. Relax.

Comments: This kriya releases stored stress and it is recommended to physically exercise after practicing. "Concentrate, meditate on yourself, feel yourself, know yourself, be yourself. Come to a solid state. You must decide. Either you control your mind and shall win, or you lose your mind and shall fail. Your reality will confront you" – Yogi Bhajan.

20 Self-Hypnosis to Experience Pratyahar

March 3, 1993

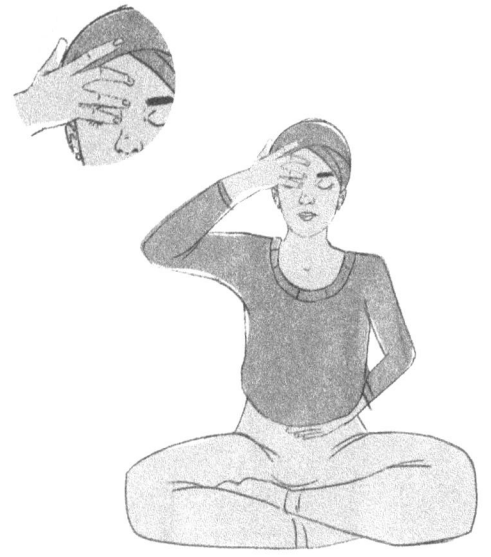

PART ONE

Sit in Easy Pose with a straight spine and apply a light Neck Lock.

Mudra: Place the left hand under clothing on the abdomen, touching the skin. With the right arm relaxed, raise the hand and place the pad of the Sun (ring) finger on the Third Eye Point, the other fingers are relaxed. Only the Sun finger and left hand are touching the body. Hold this posture steady and straight. Sit light and elevated by lifting the ribcage so that there is no weight or pressure on the liver and other abdominal organs.

Eye Focus: Closed.

Breath: Not specified.

Visualization: Imagine that you are sitting like a sage in bliss before a multitude of people. Nothing disturbs your peaceful state. Hypnotize yourself. Don't let your thoughts take you away from you. Simply be you.

Music: "God Is Within Me," by Nirinjan Kaur Khalsa was played in the class.

GOD IS WITHIN ME.
I'M DWELLING WITHIN THEE.
I HAVE NO FEAR, I SEE GOD CLEAR:
GOD IN ALL, BIG AND SMALL.
I HAVE NO FEAR, I SEE GOD CLEAR:
GOD IN ALL, BIG AND SMALL.
GOD IS WITHIN ME, ME AND GOD ARE ONE.
I'M DWELLING WITHIN THEE, GOD AND ME ARE ONE.
AS THE MOON AND SUN, SHINING ON EVERYONE.
ONE GOD ABOVE ALL,
GOD IN ALL, BIG AND SMALL.
EVERY PROBLEM OF FEAR IS SOLVED.
GOD IN ALL, BIG AND SMALL.
EVERY PROBLEM OF FEAR IS SOLVED.

CHATTR CHAKKR VARTEE, CHATTR CHAKKR BHUGATAY
SUYUMBHAV SUBHANG SARAB DAA SARAB JUGTAY
DUKAALANG PRANAASEE DAYAALANG SAROOPAY
SADAA UNG SUNGAY ABHANGANG BIBHOOTAY

Time: Meditate with the visualization for **3 ½ minutes.** Listen to the music for **10 ½ minutes** and sing it for the last **8 minutes. 22 minutes total.**

To End: Inhale deeply, suspend the breath for **15-20 seconds**, with the sensitivity of your skin feel and squeeze every part of the body from the scalp to the toes, and exhale. Repeat **2 more times.** Relax.

Comments: Without understanding self-hypnosis, you cannot live life in peace, moment to moment. Through your own power, you can protect your psyche. Nothing will bother you.

21 Body Adjustment to Eliminate Tension and Stress

March 9, 1993

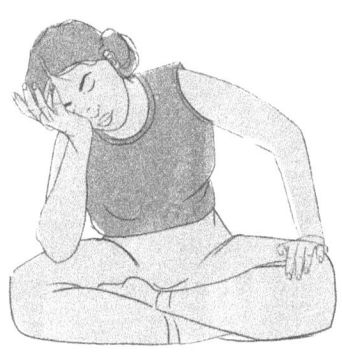

PART ONE
Sit in Easy Pose.

Mudra: Place the right elbow on the right knee and rest the right cheekbone in the palm of the right hand with the fingers loosely covering the right side of the forehead. The left hand holds the left knee with the elbow relaxed away from the body. Simply relax in this posture.

Eye Focus: Closed.

Breath: Not specified.

Music: "Guru Ram Das Lullaby"[9] was played in the class.

Time: 11 minutes.

To End: Relax the posture and assess how you feel.

Comments: This pose called Relaxing Buddha puts pressure on the liver. As you relax, the body adjusts, eliminates tension and stress and brings the sensory system into balance.

---

[9] This is a song written by Stephen Joseph, formerly Guru Shabad Singh, former member of the legendary Khalsa String Band. *"Close your eyes, it's the end of another busy day. I wouldn't be surprised if a lot of other children slept this way, with Guru Ram Das to protect them, keep them safe all through the night. Oh, Dhan Dhan Guru Ram Das, Rakho Saharanai. Meditate on Guru Nanak, may you love God with his clarity. Meditate on Guru Angad, may devotion fill your heart and set you free. Meditate on Guru Amardas, let none leave your house unfulfilled. Meditate on Guru Ram Das, Your prayers will heal the weak and the ill. Meditate on Guru Arjan, his poem is a jewel beyond all worths. Meditate on Guru Hargobind, You'll find God in heaven and on earth. Meditate on Guru Har Rai, God and you shall never be apart. Meditate on Guru Harkrishan, his sacrifice brings compassion to your heart. Meditate on Guru Teg Bahadhur, no enemy will disturb your inner peace. Meditate on Guru Gobind Singh, defend truth till your soul is released. Siri Guru Granth Sahib, may Gurbani be the love of this child's life. May it fill their hearts with wisdom and courage to bear the test of the time."*

PART TWO
Sit in Easy Pose with a straight spine and apply a light Neck Lock.

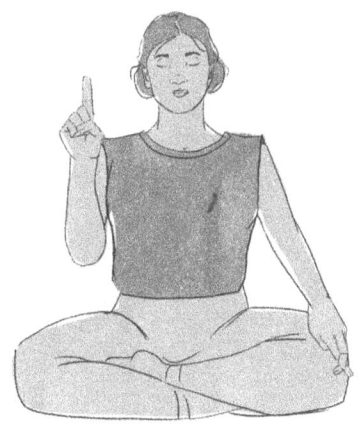

Mudra: Rest the left hand on the left knee with the Saturn (middle) finger crossed over the Jupiter (index) finger, the other two fingers locked down with the thumb, hand facing down. Relax the right elbow at the side of the body, bend the elbow with the forearm straight up and hand forward. Extend the Jupiter (index) finger straight up and the other fingers are locked down with the thumb. Move the Jupiter finger in fast small circles in a counterclockwise direction. Only the finger moves.

Eye Focus: Closed.

Breath: Not specified.

Mantra: ANG SANG WAHE GURU
(A version by Nirinjan Kaur was played in the class).

Time: 11 minutes.

To End: Inhale deeply, suspend the breath for **10 seconds**, squeeze every part of the body, keep moving the Jupiter finger, exhale, keep moving the Jupiter finger. Repeat **2 more times**. The last time, extend the suspension to **20 seconds** and move the finger as fast as possible. Relax the posture and assess how you feel.

continue on next page »

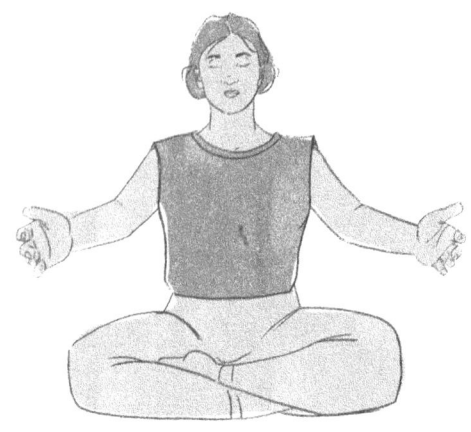

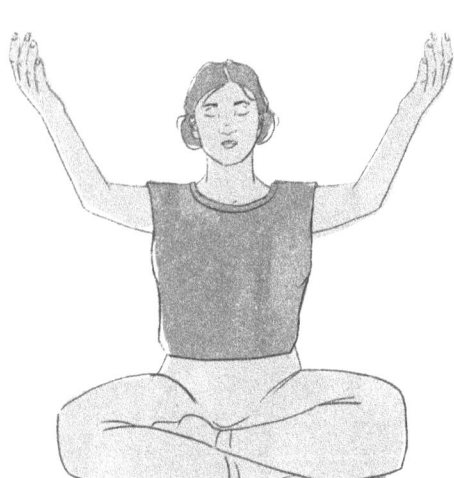

PART THREE
Sit in Easy Pose with a straight spine and apply a light Neck Lock.

Mudra: Extend your arms out in front of the body; bend the elbows so that the forearms are parallel to the ground at the level of the Solar Plexus, wider than the body. The hands face each other and are relaxed. Moving from the shoulders, arc the arms in a little and straight up above the head level, as you are pushing something up, then circle back to starting position. Push hard as you move upward.

Eye Focus: Not specified.

Breath: Not specified.

Time: 3 minutes.

To End: Inhale deeply, exhale and relax.

Comments: This posture releases old stress, so that you can live.

"You will have to survive for being you." December 1, 1992. "Time has come that you understand the depth of your life (and) that you are master of your own destiny and discipline." December 3, 1992. Basically when it boils down, you have to come to your own self with your own grips. You have to come to grips with your own life." December 8, 1992. "The highest (form of) therapy is that you should forgive yourself and others. Right on the spot, you should have an attitude of forgiveness." December 10, 1992.

22 Open to the Unknown and Know Through Intuition

March 10, 1993

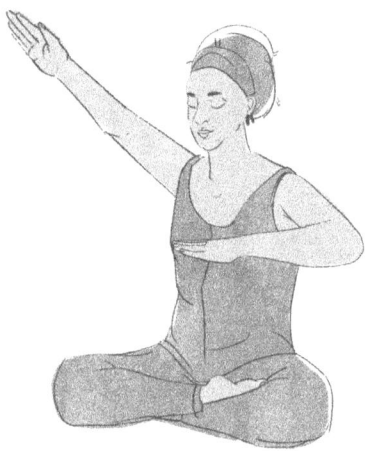

PART ONE

Sit in Easy Pose with a straight spine and apply a light Neck Lock.

Mudra: Raise the left elbow out to the side and bring the left hand in front of the Heart Center, palm facing down with the fingers together pointing to the right. The left forearm is parallel to the ground. Bring the right arm straight forward and raise it up to a 60-degree angle, palm facing down and fingers together. Keep the right arm straight, elbow stretched.

Eye Focus: Closed.

Breath: One Minute Breath (**20 seconds** inhale, **20 seconds** suspend, **20 seconds** exhale).

Mental Focus: Feel the divine presence within or feel the presence of the deity you believe in surrounding you.

Time: 11 minutes.

To End: Inhale deeply, suspend the breath for **15 seconds**, squeeze the body and spread any discomfort throughout the body, exhale. Repeat **2 more times**, holding the last breath for **25 seconds**. Relax the posture and move the body – hands, shoulders, and rib cage – for **1-2 minutes**.

Comments: Become aware of any discomfort in your body and allow it to happen. The discomfort affects the pineal gland and the stretch in the armpit balances the sympathetic, parasympathetic and enteric nervous systems, which gives you support to face the pain in life. You may play an uplifting music or mantra to help you keep up with the posture. ("Aadays Tisay Aadays," by Nirinjan Kaur was played in the original class).

PART TWO

Sit in Easy Pose with a straight spine and apply a light Neck Lock.

Mudra: Extend both arms straight out in front of the body parallel to the ground, palms pressed together, with thumbs crossed and fingers pointing forward. Strongly whistle a song of your choice. The stronger, the better it will work.

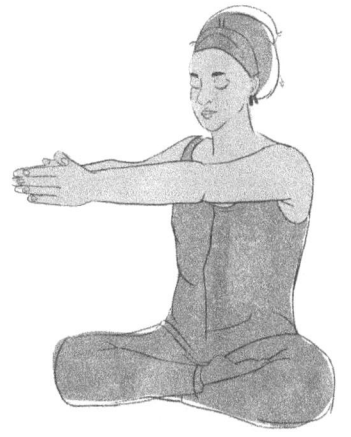

Eye Focus: Closed.

Breath: Not specified.

Time: 7 minutes.

continue on next page »

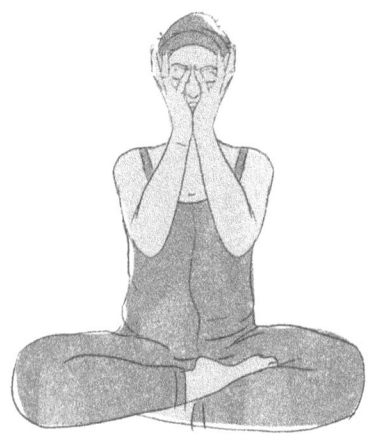

PART THREE
Remain in Easy Pose with a straight spine and apply a light Neck Lock.

Mudra: Raise both arms up with the elbows out to the sides. Place the hands in Lotus Mudra in front of the face with the base of the palms at the level of the tip of the nose. Hold the hands firm and steady and completely relax the rest of the body. For Lotus Mudra, begin by bringing the hands together in Prayer Pose. Keeping the base of the palms, tips of the thumbs and Mercury (little) fingers touching, open the hands and spread the fingers like a flower opening. No other part of the hands or fingers touch.

Eye Focus: Closed.

Breath: Not specified.

Time: 3 minutes.

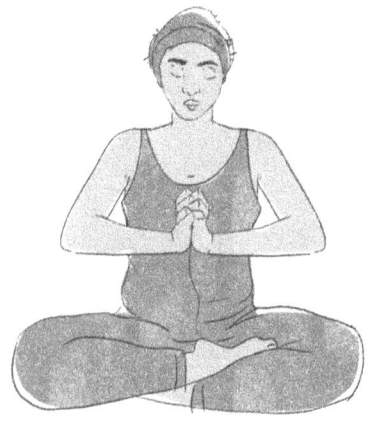

To End: Bring the hands in front of the Heart Center, interlock the fingers. The elbows are out to the sides, forearms parallel to the ground. Inhale, suspend the breath for **10 seconds** and press the palms together as hard as you can, exhale. Repeat **2 more times**. Relax and talk to each other if you are practicing in a class, or talk to yourself, if practicing alone.

Comments: The duality of the tension of holding the mudra and the total relaxation of the rest of the body recharges the body's energy.

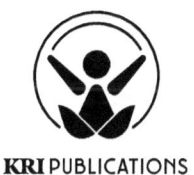

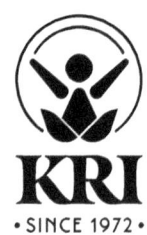

A Kundalini Yoga Global Community
KUNDALINIRESEARCHINSTITUTE.ORG

www.ingramcontent.com/pod-product-compliance
Lightning Source LLC
Chambersburg PA
CBHW080402030426
42334CB00024B/2966